# FORECASTING USE OF HEALTH SERVICES

## A Provider's Guide

Robin Scott MacStravic, Ph.D.
Vice President for Planning and Marketing
Health and Hospital Services
Bellevue, Washington

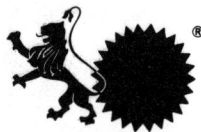

AN ASPEN PUBLICATION®
Aspen Systems Corporation
Rockville, Maryland
Royal Tunbridge Wells
1984

Library of Congress Cataloging in Publication Data

MacStravic, Robin E.
Forecasting use of health services.


"An Aspen publication."
Includes bibliographies and index.
1. Medical care — Utilization — Forecasting. 2. Health facilities —
Utilization — Forecasting. 3. Medical care — Utilization —
Mathematical models. 4. Health facilities—Utilization—
Mathematical models. I. Title.
RA410.5.M328      1984      338.4'73621      84-6333
ISBN: 0-89443-857-3

Publisher: John R. Marozsan
Associate Publisher: Jack W. Knowles, Jr.
Editor-in-Chief: Mike Brown
Executive Managing Editor: Margot G. Raphael
Managing Editor: M. Eileen Higgins
Editorial Services: Martha Sasser
Printing and Manufacturing: Debbie Collins

Library of Congress Catalog Card Number: 84-6333
ISBN: 0-89443-857-3

*Printed in the United States of America*

1   2   3   4   5

# Table of Contents

# Preface

This book is intended as a guide to forecasting techniques that can be used to estimate future use of health services. These techniques can be used for many other purposes, but those discussed in this book are most likely to be used for health services. The author has personally used or critically examined all the techniques. Although this book offers the author's personal biases regarding the strengths and limitations of specific techniques, such biases are based on practical experience. Readers whose biases differ from the author's should find useful guidance in the selection and employment of available techniques, even if the author's recommendations are ignored.

With the advent of microprocessors and increasing sophistication of portable calculators, almost anyone can employ complex forecasting techniques. What makes a good forecast, however, is not the complexity of the technique or the quantity of data used. Rather it is the quality of the thinking that goes into the forecasting process. Increasing dependence on gadgetry can misdirect forecasting efforts and produce results that are judged by the impressiveness of the technique rather than the likelihood of its result. Forecasters and decision makers who evaluate forecasts must keep in mind the subjective assumptions and choices that go into employing a forecasting technique as well as the analysis and calculations that actually produce the forecast.

One traditional response to the development of new technologies that substitute machine for man is to attack the machines, as the Luddites did in England early in the nineteenth century. Another, equally unfortunate, response is to embrace the new technology as necessarily better. The fact that computers can instantaneously calculate uncountable sums, remainders, products, and quotients should not lead to their automatic adoption in forecasting. It is even more true in forecasting than in other computer uses that garbage in equals garbage out. The quality of the thought and instructions more than that of the data will dictate whether computer-generated forecasts turn out well.

Any forecasting discussion must balance the need for informed analytic thinking with the reality that the future cannot be precisely known. It is all too common for health care planners and managers to shrug off forecasting with the conclusion that nothing can be accurately estimated more than one or two years ahead. This is a perfectly valid conclusion if *accuracy* is defined narrowly and applied rigidly. The future is subject only to earnest and careful conjecture, to informed speculation, not to the sort of quantitative calculation that the past permits.

On the other hand all planning decisions and many management decisions are based on estimates of the future. It would be cavalier to treat the future as a blank space about which not even reasonable guesses can be made. The purpose of this book is to present and examine state-of-the-art thinking relative to making reasonable guesses about future health services utilization. It is based on the conviction that better decisions can be made based on reasonable guesses than on deliberate ignorance.

In many cases a better decision will result if forecasters can promise even the direction in which utilization will change. In others an estimate within plus or minus 10 or 20 percent may serve perfectly well. In my own professional practice I have generally managed to come within 5 percent of the future in immediate forecasts (up to one year), within 10 percent in intermediate forecasts (up to five years), and within 20 percent in longer-term forecasts. This degree of accuracy has been sufficient for almost every situation where a forecast was called for.

In decision making, as opposed to science, it is unnecessary to be right in the sense of high precision and accuracy. It is necessary only to be close enough for the decision to turn out well. The forecasting techniques presented in this book, and the discussions of their application to health services use, should aid decision makers in producing more useful forecasts and more effective decisions.

The book is divided into six parts designed to cover the use of forecasts as well as techniques for producing them. Part I covers the forecasting context, examining the reasons for making forecasts in the first place and how those reasons should influence the choice of a technique or approach. Individual chapters discuss the exact forecast required to meet the needs of decision makers, the context and technical choices available to forecasters, and the manner in which selections should be made among alternative techniques.

Part II addresses the most common quantitative forecasting techniques. All are categorized as projection techniques in that they project the future as a continuation of some pattern of utilization change or stability identified in the past. Individual chapters discuss linear extrapolations, autocorrelation, and analytical techniques. One chapter is devoted to a specific marketing projection technique based on product life cycle and innovation adoption patterns.

Part III covers prediction techniques. These forecasting approaches predict health services utilization as a function of one or more other factors. Predictive factors are typically deemed independent variables, with health services utilization the dependent variable whose future depends on what happens to one or more independent variables. Specific chapters address the causal context underlying all prediction techniques, as well as selected examples of predictions based on population, health system, and environmental variables and techniques incorporating multiple predictive variables.

Part IV covers prospection techniques, i.e., forecasts that merely look to the future rather than rely on the past. Such techniques may be purely subjective and speculative or involve systematic analysis of the dynamics affecting utilization of health services. Individual chapters address naive approaches, which can be independent of data and analysis, and analytic approaches which are based on identified change factors. An examination of ways of combining forecasting techniques, segment forecasts, or multiple forecasts rounds out this discussion.

Part V addresses a common and important forecasting challenge, the need to anticipate patterns of variation in use of health services over time as well as total volumes. Most of the analysis in this part is based on original work by the author and is specific to health services. Individual chapters address fluctuations in the use of health services within one year and variations in total utilization from year to year. The applications of variation forecasts in making capacity and operational decisions are specifically addressed. A method for using known variation patterns to forecast utilization is presented.

Part VI completes the book with systematic discussions of the uses of forecasts in planning and management decisions. Forecasts are intended to be useful, educated guesses about the future, with the emphasis on useful. Individual chapters discuss using forecasts in making decisions and forecasting the demand for a new service.

This book is written for people who have no training in statistics and those who have substantial statistical knowledge and skills. Wherever possible, it incorporates forecasting techniques that can be used by anyone with a basic mathematical aptitude. Those with statistical skills will undoubtedly derive more from discussions of forecasting techniques involving statistical concepts and tools. No reader should skip any chapter, however, even though some of the discussion may require familiarity with statistics to be fully appreciated. A glossary is provided at the end of the book to assist the reader with the language of forecasting.

Robin Scott MacStravic
Mercer Island, Washington

# Acknowledgments

This book is dedicated to the National Center for Health Statistics, to the Applied Statistical Training Institutes, and to Moshman Associates of Washington, D.C., which challenged me in 1980 to develop a five-day workshop on forecasting the use of health services. At the time I certainly didn't know five days' worth of forecasting to discuss. This challenge forced me to pore through the literature on forecasting in general, on the unique models and applications appropriate to health services, and on actual forecasts used in health care.

I sought out planners, budgeters, administrators, and other forecasters in health care organizations to discover their interests and techniques in forecasting. The workshops that I conducted in 1981 and 1982 provided additional opportunities to discuss forecasting demand for health care with practitioners. I can only hope that what I was forced to learn in order to teach is adequately reflected in this book.

Special thanks must go to my secretary, Sue Scott, who after coping with my verbal ramblings during the day was willing to type this manuscript in her spare time.

# Part I

# The Forecasting Context

Although this book is intended as a practical, do-it-yourself guide to the selection and application of forecasting techniques, some discussion of the forecasting context is necessary. Forecasting techniques are not employed in a vacuum; hence their environment should be taken into account in considering which technique to employ and in determining how to use it. If the proper contextual basis for a forecast is not carefully developed, the forecast will probably be wasted.

Chapter 1 discusses the task of determining exactly what is to be forecast and why. Because the book focuses on forecasting health services utilization, part of the answer to what is being forecast is already determined. Questions remain about aspects of utilization, time period, area, and population. To answer these questions, it is critical that the reasons for developing a forecast and its intended use be specified. In other words in planning a forecast, like any other planning task, it is essential to answer in advance who, what, where, when, how, and why. In forecasting, all the $W$ questions are answered in order to decide how.

Chapter 2 discusses the basic choices regarding forecasting process and output, which determine what techniques to consider. The time frame of a forecast addresses the major point of the period of time's utilization to be forecast. The choice between a naive versus causal approach to forecasting addresses the question of whether the forecaster can and will ask why utilization of health services occurs and changes over time. The option of using a passive or interventional approach to forecasting asks whether the forecaster is able or willing to interfere in the dynamics that affect health services utilization or will simply try to estimate what will happen to developments beyond control.

Chapter 3 discusses specific criteria and procedures for selecting among alternative forecasting techniques. The worth of a technique is measured in terms of the precision, confidence, and acceptability of the forecast output, the specific utilization information estimate for the future. The cost of using a technique relates to the financial costs of data, analysis, time, and effort plus the complexity of the technique and its potential for producing needed estimates in time for use in decision making. As in all choices, the worth of a technique relative to its costs represents the best basis for selection.

**Chapter 1**

# What to Forecast and Why

It is by no means trivial to ask exactly what is to be forecast. Because this book addresses the task of forecasting the use of health services, the question is partly answered. In order to identify forecasting alternatives, select and implement the best choice, the exact nature and extent of what is to be forecast, over what period of time, must be specified. The earlier and more precisely the output of the forecast can be specified, the better the task can be performed.

## DECISION CONTEXT

To identify exactly what is to be forecast, it is essential to begin with the specification of the decision to be made. Unless idle curiosity instigates an attempt to forecast the use of health services, some decisions will be made based on that forecast. In a budgeting situation a forecast of utilization may be a basis for predicting revenues and expenditures, staffing plans, or supplies purchases. A resources decision to determine how large a facility to build or how much equipment to buy would be based on anticipated utilization as would a "go" versus "no-go" decision regarding a new program.

The exact nature of the decisions to be made should be the first step in any forecasting process. The specific type of information needed, the necessity of making a forecast credible, the period over which utilization must be forecast—all are conditioned on the decision to be made. A process that produces the forecast first, then moves on to seeing what kinds of decisions can be made from it, tends to stretch the value and usefulness of the forecast beyond its potential. By specifying in careful detail the precise decision to be made, the forecasting process takes on a necessary and practical focus likely to be missed otherwise.

3

## SUCCESS CRITERIA

Once the decision context is specified, the next step follows logically. In order to know exactly what to forecast, it is necessary to know what aspects of utilization will determine whether the decisions to be made turn out successfully. What criteria will be used to evaluate the decision after it is made and implemented? Given those criteria, what features of utilization over what period will cause good versus bad outcomes on those criteria?

If the decision to be made is a go versus no-go or any other type of discrete decision, identifiable aspects of utilization should suggest the best decision. It may be the number of people using a service, visits, admissions, patient days, or prescriptions or any other numerical measure of utilization. It might also be the mix of patients; the proportions that have certain conditions; who will pay full charges, restricted costs, or nothing; males and females; children and adults; or many other possible attributes of the users of services that will determine whether a program succeeds.

If the choice is to be made among competing locations for a new program, the relative utilization levels expected at each site would be critical in deciding. The attributes of users as well as the sheer volume of use may tip the scales in favor of one alternative versus another. The precision of a forecast in such circumstances might be satisfactory if it merely enables determining which site promises a clearly superior pattern of utilization. In deciding to go with a new program, the precision of the forecast required may be enough to tell if and when the program will reach break-even level.

In forecasting as well as in estimating the past or present, two criteria are important but distinct and are often confused in discussions. *Precision* refers to how close to a specific number a forecast is. A utilization forecast that guesses total patient visits at 5,000 plus or minus 1,000, or plus or minus 20 percent, is not precise. One that guesses 5,000 plus or minus 5, or plus or minus .1 percent, is extremely precise. Precision is a major consideration in forecasting because a range is the most likely output of any forecasting process. If the range is too wide, it doesn't help to make the decision. It can never be too narrow, as long as it is correct.

*Accuracy* refers to how close a forecast is to actual future utilization. Unlike precision, accuracy can never be determined until the future happens. We all want our forecasts to be accurate, but accuracy is by definition a retrospective concept applied to a prospective process. A technique that has produced admirably accurate forecasts may be considered an accurate *technique* based on past performance. The forecast that it produces, however, can be judged accurate only when compared to the future. If a utilization forecast results in a no-go decision, its accuracy can never be determined.

To know what aspects of health services utilization will determine whether a decision turns out successfully, it is essential to know what constitutes success within the organization making the decision. Ideally, explicit success criteria have been identified by the organization as part of its strategic and operational planning. If so, success criteria relevant to the specific decisions under consideration can be selected. If not, an earnest attempt should be made to identify criteria that can be used for the decision. These should be closely related to the implicit success criteria of the organization and may serve as the basis for making them more explicit. The more explicitly and completely the success criteria pertinent to a decision can be identified, the more useful and effective a forecast can be made.

**Categories**

Based on the author's experience since 1964 in consulting with and working in health care organizations on strategic planning and marketing issues, success criteria tend to fall into eight categories:

1. financial health
2. image or reputation
3. service appropriateness and adequacy
4. quality of professional care
5. efficiency
6. resources
7. contribution to the community and the health care system
8. satisfaction of all who deal with the hospital

*Financial health* is a logical starting place, but unless the organization has a total profit orientation, it is not necessarily the most important success criterion. Health care organizations may have explicit, minimal expectations for "profit" or net contribution to reserves on an annual basis. They may not wish to make more than this minimum, however. Some minimum financial health is considered necessary in order for a provider to do its job, but bigger and better financial returns are not necessarily treated as ends in themselves.

Utilization affects financial health in a variety of ways. The sheer volume of the use of specific services affects expenditure levels and revenues. The types of patients using services in terms of diagnosis and acuity level affect the amount of care required, hence costs of care, plus charges and payment levels under diagnosis related group (DRG) pricing schemes. The mix of patients by payment source greatly affects revenues, given the differences in actual income expected from privately insured, governmentally insured, self-pay, and charity patients. The more that can be accurately forecast about which and how many people will use which and how many services, the better the organization can make budget and program decisions, especially under prospective payment.

*Image* covers how people perceive the provider that cares for them, what they know or believe to be true about it, and how they feel toward it. In contrast to financial health, where ample data are available in the provider's own records, image normally requires a systematic survey of community residents, referral area physicians, industries, potential donors, lenders, etc. Moreover no industry standards cover what a provider's image should be.

The provider's image may be considered important for its own sake (its intrinsic value) or chiefly for its effect on other success criteria such as utilization and financial health (its instrumental value). Each provider must decide how it values its image as well as what sort of image it wishes and how much it is willing to commit to achieving a desired image.

Image can be a major influence on the three factors that determine utilization of a specific provider. *Retention* is the proportion of the local market that seeks care among local providers. It is greatly affected by the extent to which local populations feel that local services are as good as or better than opportunities elsewhere. *Inflow* is the amount of use of local providers by people from other markets. It is determined by the extent to which people feel that local providers are better than providers in the home market and as good as other distant options. *Competitive market share* is the proportion of combined retention and inflow that is captured by a specific provider. It is determined by the competitive distinctions that the provider is perceived to have over other local providers.

*Service* reflects the extent to which the provider offers the types and amounts of services that best fit the community's need and the provider's capabilities. Although this criterion is an objective measure, the standards to which the provider's service mix would be compared are entirely subjective. Are community residents satisfied that the provider offers the correct set of services? Are regulatory and reimbursement organizations satisfied? Are the provider's professional employees also satisfied? Does everyone feel that the provider offers comprehensive or at least well-coordinated services that respond to the needs of the community? Is the provider satisfied that it is offering everything that it is capable of and only those services that it performs well?

Decisions as to whether to offer or continue any given service must be made on the basis of anticipated utilization. The need for care means the number of people who will potentially use a given service. Decisions on offering the service should be made based on utilization that will occur, however, rather than what might theoretically be needed. Because of the impact of utilization patterns on the success of any service decision, it should be the most important, if not sole, basis on which service decisions are made.

*Quality* of care is easily one of the most important success criteria, although one of the most difficult to measure. It can be addressed in objective terms by examining the resources used in patient care, the activities of patient care, or its outcomes. It can be measured subjectively by asking patients and professionals how they perceive the provider's quality of care. It may be measured indirectly by monitoring incident reports, malpractice suits, complaints, etc.

Quality is influenced by utilization in key ways. Some minimum level of utilization is needed to justify the appropriate personnel and equipment, for example. Minimum levels of utilization are required in many cases to maintain skill levels of those providing services. On the other hand utilization levels that overtax the capacity of space, equipment, and personnel cause reductions in quality. Forecasts of utilization should help in making decisions about whether appropriate quality can be maintained and what resources are necessary to do so.

*Efficiency* relates the utilization of the provider's services to the resources used or available to provide care. It is intended to reflect how much the provider does with its resources compared to its capacity for rendering service. Efficiency and productivity measures are almost always relationship measures: rates or ratios compared to the provider's own capacity, industrial standards, budgeted expectations, or financial requirements. Efficiency is a function of marketing as well as management success because it is so directly affected by the provider's ability to attract and retain customers, as well as its management of its resources.

Efficiency is essentially the extent to which the organization's resources are used at close to their capacity. Utilization would be the numerator in any calculation of efficiency, with capacity or service potential in the denominator. Decisions regarding short- and long-term capacity are made in anticipation of utilization. If forecasts are in error, substantial adjustments may be required to achieve desired efficiency with unexpected utilization levels.

*Resource measures* cover qualitative and quantitative adequacy and appropriateness of the provider's resources: its land, facilities, equipment, human resources, supplies, and information. The intention is to reflect whether the provider has enough but not too much of exactly what it needs to carry out its basic mission and to achieve desired performance relative to other success criteria. Resource measures may be intrinsically valued or rated entirely on the basis of their instrumental impact on other measures such as costs (financial health), efficiency, services, and image.

Resource decisions are made based on utilization anticipated and are evaluated based on utilization actually experienced. Use of each program's space, equipment, and personnel should be as close as possible to what was expected when decisions regarding those resources were made. Space and equipment decisions are particularly difficult to adjust if utilization is significantly more or less than anticipated. Hence accurate forecasts of utilization, by specific program or even specific resource, are needed to make appropriate resource decisions.

*Contribution* is easily the most difficult success criterion to define, though not necessarily the most difficult to measure after being well defined. It is intended to reflect the extent to which the community served by the provider is and perhaps perceives itself to be benefiting from the provider's existence and the way it operates. Any ways in which the provider feels community residents are better off because of what it does, as well as any ways in which the community perceives itself to be better off, are proper items for inclusion in this category. In the broadest sense, contribution is the reason that the provider is in business and represents the most intrinsically valuable aspect of its success.

Specific measures that might be used to reflect a hospital's contribution for example, could be

- the level of health knowledge of local citizens resulting from hospital-sponsored educational and public information programs (e.g., cardio-pulmonary resuscitation (CPR) training, parent education, death and dying programs)
- the number of health professionals trained by the hospital (e.g., nurses, residents, and interns)
- any mental or physical health status improvements attributable to hospital programs (e.g., poison information, stress or pain management, exercise, nutrition)
- any cost reductions, i.e., local cost per capita for hospital care, attributable to the organization's own efforts
- the financial and employment contribution made by the hospital to the local community

Typically the hospital would focus not only on the reality of each of these measures but also on the extent to which they are recognized and appreciated by the community, i.e., reflected in image measures.

*Satisfaction* covers the extent to which the expectations of everyone who deals with the provider are met. It is by definition a subjective criterion, though it might be reflected in objective measures; employee satisfaction might be reflected in turnover rates, for example. It is a success criterion that is directly related to a number of others, such as contribution, quality, and efficiency, and may be valued only for its instrumental impact or at least partly for its own intrinsic value. It may include the satisfaction of trustees, administrators, medical staff, visitors, employees, physicians, suppliers—everyone who interacts with the organization.

Satisfaction of patients obviously is a major factor in affecting utilization levels. Satisfied patients should return for additional care and even recommend the satisfactory provider to their acquaintances, while dissatisfied patients will do the opposite. Utilization levels also significantly affect employee satisfaction. Low utilization undermines morale as well as makes it difficult to retain confidence in employment. Excessive utilization for given staffing levels threatens quality and places unwelcome stress on employees.

## Implications

Two major implications of explicit success criteria should be clear from this discussion. First, the great number of such criteria reflects the wide scope and complexity of the ways that health care providers define success. A major task in using success criteria is to select a number sufficient to provide the needed information but small enough to be manageable. Approximately 15 to 25 explicit measures are all that can be handled on a regular basis. For specific problems or programs, special subsets of measures may be used on a temporary basis.

The second implication lies in the fact that roughly half of the useful measures can be employed only through surveys of subjective feelings. Provider records can usually supply the other half, but image, service, quality, resources, contribution, and satisfaction are almost bound to include, if not rely on, the results of surveys for effective measurement.

Although each organization has its own success criteria, those most likely to be involved when basing a decision on a utilization forecast fall in the financial, quality, efficiency, and contribution categories. The combined effect of future utilization on one or more of these criteria in most cases determines whether a given decision turns out well. Therefore, what should be forecast are those quantitative and qualitative aspects of health services utilization that produce the combined effect.

In any decision situation how and to what extent utilization affects finances, image, service, quality, efficiency, resources, contribution, and satisfaction, i.e., all the success criteria likely to apply to a health organization, should be considered. It may be the level of utilization, its sheer volume, its timing, its need-of-care characteristics, its variability, or some combination that determines the overall impact. Whatever features of utilization determine the levels of performance or success achieved through a given decision should be the precise features of utilization forecast before that decision is made. If the relationship between utilization characteristics and success criteria outcomes are well understood and identified in advance, the importance of utilization and the different impacts of foreseeable utilization levels can be determined easily as forecasts are made. The extent of precision and confidence required of a forecast is determined by the nature and extent of the impact of utilization levels on success criteria.

## WHO, WHERE, AND WHEN

The *what* question in forecasting utilization necessarily includes the *who* and *where* questions as well. People use health services (or animals do, if you're in veterinary services). Therefore, the people who can, should, and will use the services must be immediately specified as a basis for estimating utilization. Even if a naive forecasting technique is employed, knowledge of the users of services is essential in judging the validity of assumptions intrinsic to the technique. The size of the population served, its demographic and psychographic characteristics, and its present behavior are important in estimating its future health services utilization behavior.

Where health services will be used involves who will be using them and where they will go for them. Forecasting the use of a specific provider of services, for example, requires first estimating how people will use health services in general. Once their total use of care is forecast, the extent to which they will seek it at a given provider (the provider's market share) must be estimated. The characteristics of the provider and of competing alternatives must be considered in forecasting market share.

The *when* question in forecasting includes both the period over which forecasts are required and the deadline when the forecast is needed. Time frames for forecasting are discussed in Chapter 2. The timing of the forecast is a critical consideration for evaluating which technique can be used (Chapter 3).

## SUMMARY

The first essential step in forecasting health services utilization is to identify explicitly and precisely what is to be forecast. To carry out this step, the decisions to be made based on the forecast must be specified as clearly and completely as possible. Then the success criteria or performance outcomes that dictate whether that decision is correct, i.e., the criteria that are used to judge it retrospectively, are identified. Finally, the nature and extent of impact expected from alternative features of utilization (i.e., total volume, type, timing, variability) are identified.

With this context established, the specific utilization information necessary to making an informed decision is identified. That is precisely the utilization information that should be forecast, no more and no less. The time frame of information needed, its precision, and confidence are determined based on the decision-making context thus established. Without such a context the value of utilization forecasts and their usefulness in making decisions are left to chance.

---

**Annotated Bibliography**

**Cantor, J.** *Pragmatic Forecasting.* New York: American Management Association, 1971.
   Discusses the uses to which forecasts are put and how the application of forecasts in making decisions determines which techniques are appropriate.

**Cleverly, W.** "Profitability Analysis in the Hospital Industry." *Health Services Research* 13, no. 1 (Spring 1978): 16.
   Discusses the use of utilization forecasts in deciding how to invest resources.

**Gardner, E., and McLaughlin, C.** "Forecasting: A Cost Control Tool for Health Managers." *Health Care Management Review* 5, no. 3 (Summer 1980): 31.
   Describes how forecasts of utilization can be used to minimize operating and capital expenditures.

**Harrington, M.** "Forecasting Areawide Demand for Health Care Services: A Critical Review of Major Techniques and Their Application." *Inquiry* 14, no. 3 (September 1977): 254.
   Discusses the use of forecasts of utilization in the areawide planning process and the importance of knowing the purpose for forecasting.

**Kretchmar, C.** "How to Forecast Your Rates—Without Guessing," *Hospital Financial Management* 6, no. 7 (July 1976): 44.
   Discusses how to use utilization forecasts to determine hospital charges.

**Mitchell, F.** "Anticipation versus Results: An Approach to Improved Program Forecasting," *American Journal of Health Planning* 3, no. 2 (April 1978): 7.
   Discusses the use and importance of utilization forecasts in the planning process.

**Raedels, A., and Mason, J.** "Forecasting an Ill Wind: Forecasting Physician Requirements for a University Health Care Centre." *Proceedings of the American Institute of Decision Sciences Annual Meeting,* November 1978, p. 25.

**Wensley, R.** "Principles of Useful Market Forecasting." *Management Decision* 17, no. 4 (1979): 295.
   Discusses the importance of market forecasting to the decision-making process.

# Chapter 2

# Forecasting Choices

Numerous choices must be made once the what and why of utilization forecasting have been determined. Before selecting a specific technique, or a set of techniques, for producing a forecast, decisions must be made as to the time frame over which utilization is to be forecast, the type of forecasting technique that is applicable, and whether an interventionist versus passive approach is more appropriate. These decisions greatly facilitate the selection of the proper forecasting techniques and significantly narrow the range of options that even need to be considered. The data requirements and availability in any situation also influence available choices.

## TIME FRAMES

The period over which a demand for health services is to be forecast is a function of two factors: lead time and duration for the decisions that are to be made based on the forecast. Lead time refers to time needed to implement a decision, the delay in response peculiar to any specific decision. Duration refers to the time during which the decision, once implemented, continues to interact with demand to affect the organization's performance. Lead time indicates the beginning of the period for which a forecast is needed, and duration indicates the extent or length of the period.

### Lead Time

The time needed to implement a decision varies widely, depending on the type of decisions to be made. Assigning personnel to one activity or service versus another may require a lead time of a few hours to a day. Acquiring temporary staff to cover a period of peak demand may require

24 hours, or more than one day's lead time. Recruiting a new physician may take a number of months, perhaps a year. Purchasing major equipment is likely to require an anticipation of demand a year or more ahead. Building a new facility or expanding current space may take three to five years.

The nature of the decision and the forecast itself work to create different kinds of lead time even when the same type of decision is to be made. It may be possible to add staff temporarily with little lead time if the forecast indicates increasing demand, although it takes a week or longer to arrange for temporary layoffs or vacations if the forecast indicates declining demand. If the reactions to the forecast can vary, then the lead time can vary. A decision to close a wing of a facility or even to convert unused facility space for other purposes, in anticipation of declining or continuing low demand, can probably be implemented in several months. A commitment to add a wing or office space may take years, considering the financing, planning, and regulatory factors involved.

Not only the direction but the extent of demand forecast can affect the lead time. If the forecast indicates a mild increase in demand, various expedients may be employed to increase hospital capacity mildly. Private hospital rooms may be converted to semiprivate, or surgery may be switched to a six-day rather than five-day schedule. A clinic may slightly expand its hours or add another day to accommodate mildly increasing demand. Dramatic increases are more likely to require capital expenditures, which in turn necessitates more lead time. The expedients may be used in the interim, but the lead time necessary for such expenditures is likely to be far longer than the lead time necessary for modest changes.

Thus the lead time appropriate for a forecast is only partly predictable. It may be anticipated that a forecast of next year's demand is all that is needed for modest decisions. Yet that forecast might represent such a dramatic change in demand that more significant responses become necessary, but with a lead time greater than one year. In such a case the decision will be late, with potentially disastrous consequences on performance.

It is generally a good idea to forecast as far ahead as the maximum lead time necessary for the types of responses likely to be needed. The hospital should always have its eye on what demand is likely to be five years ahead in case a dramatic change is in sight and a major response will be needed. Otherwise the future may sneak up on the organization with a dramatic change in demand and the organization may not have the ability to respond promptly because of lead time.

### Correction Point

The lead time required to make a response is not the only factor that should be recognized in timing a forecast. Its correction or adjustment point should also be identified. For any particular decision there is likely to be a point in time before implementation when it can be reversed or modified. A decision to add temporary staff may be cancelable with 12 hours' notice, for example, even though its lead time is 24 hours. A commitment to buy a new piece of equipment may be cancelable until 30 days before delivery. A decision to build a new facility may be reversible up to two years before its scheduled opening, even though its lead time is five years.

Typically the ability to adjust or alter a decision is limited. If on further reflection demand seems to be going up faster than anticipated, it may not be possible to increase the size of an addition to capacity without more lead time. If the forecast seems overly optimistic, however, expanding capacity may be subject to cancellation or delay with relatively little lead time. If there is a later point in time when a previous decision can be changed, a revised or at least reconsidered forecast should be made at that point.

**Duration**

The length of time in which a decision endures is subject to more variability than lead time. A decision to stop elective admissions because of high occupancy and expected emergency admissions could last as briefly as a few hours or as long as a number of weeks. Hiring temporary personnel for peak demand periods may entail a commitment of a day, a week, or more. Recruiting professionals may involve a contract covering a year or more. Purchasing equipment may burden the organization with its costs for many years, where a lease may involve only a single year. Deciding to renovate a building may increase fixed costs for 10 to 15 years, where a new facility might involve a duration of 20 or 30 years.

The forecast of demand should indicate whether a long-duration decision is warranted. A confident expectation of continuing high utilization or greater increases in demand would justify an enduring commitment. A forecast of a short-term surge in demand followed by decline or return to normal would suggest some temporary expedient. In either case the expected general pattern of demand, over the entire time when the decision and its consequences would be in effect, should be incorporated in the decision making.

*Correction Point*

There is a correction point with respect to duration also. Short of the expected or normal duration for a particular decision, there is likely to be a point when the situation may be altered accordingly if demand proves other than expected. Personnel already hired and working may be reassigned or laid off. Equipment purchased may be sold; unused facilities may be converted to other uses. As long as some reasonable use can be made of capital or personnel assets within their expected, useful lives, correction or adaptation may mitigate the effects of an incorrect decision or an overly optimistic forecast.

There is likely to be a limited extent to which most decisions may be corrected, once implemented, short of their expected duration. Personnel may have to be retrained before they can be reassigned; facilities may have to be renovated substantially. Once it is realized that forecasts were in error, correction may take months or years to achieve. Certificate-of-need approval may be necessary in order to eliminate a service that has proven unsuccessful in attracting demand. Union contracts may restrict reassignment of personnel. There must be some useful purpose to which assets can be applied for a correction to represent a positive adaptation to unexpected demand levels.

## IMPLICATIONS FOR FORECASTING

Combining lead time and duration, the key period for which demand should be forecast is the period from the earliest point when a decision could be implemented (current period plus lead time) to the earliest point when a decision, once implemented, could be corrected (decision point plus correction time). Demand for this period should be estimated with all reasonable care, once for making the decision, then again at the latest possible correction point before implementation. A third series of running forecasts should be made once the decision has been implemented, just far enough ahead to equal the earliest possible correction point after implementation.

These forecasts represent different periods of time for different decisions, and different periods of time for the three points at which forecasts are made. Because of these differences, it is likely and appropriate that a variety of forecasting techniques be used. The choice of techniques then determines the amount of time in the past for which data are to be collected.

### Naive versus Causal Techniques

A standard division among forecasting techniques is based on the distinction between naive and causal approaches to estimating the future. A *naive* technique makes no attempt to incorporate any understanding of or information about *why* health services utilization is what it is at any point in time. A *causal* technique implicitly or explicitly incorporates such understanding and information. All forecasting techniques are either naive or causal, and the distinction provides an early and significant choice relative to available techniques.

*Naive* techniques treat future utilization as a function of past and present utilization. They are almost always quantitative, objective techniques in which past or present utilization is analyzed through some mathematical function. This function is then used to estimate the future. As objective, mathematical techniques, they may seem more scientific or at least unbiased than some other options, but they are not. The selection of a naive technique automatically builds in the bias of the technique itself, which is often not even recognized. (A Delphi technique is usually naive, though it can be used causally, and is an example of a quantitative, *subjective* forecasting technique. See Chapter 12.)

Because naive techniques are naive, that is, require no knowledge of or information about the causes of utilization, they are usually simpler to employ than causal techniques. Some sophisticated and complex forecasting techniques, however, are absolutely naive. The Box-Jenkins and Autoregressive Integrated Moving Averages (ARIMA) techniques are computer-based approaches that employ substantial data bases on past utilization to project the future. Neither requires or employs information about the causes that underlie past utilization patterns or affect future utilization. (Neither is described and discussed in detail in this book because they are not capable of a do-it-yourself application.)

Naive techniques are also a little riskier than causal alternatives in most cases. Because they don't address factors that have caused changes in utilization, they can't incorporate any differences in how such factors might behave in the future. They rely on the usually unstated assumption that whatever dynamics have produced the patterns of utilization observed in the past and present will continue to operate unchanged. Such an assumption should always be identified and examined before a naive technique is considered. There may be good reason to accept such an assumption or there may be no choice, but it should always be made clear that naive techniques rest on this basic assumption.

Because it must be assumed that no changes in the dynamics affecting utilization will occur, naive techniques generally are limited in application. They should be used only for short time frames because changes in dynamics are not only possible but likely in intermediate and long time frames. They should also be used only in essentially stable or unpredictable situations. Utilization by large populations (major cities, states, etc.) tends to follow patterns much more than utilization by smaller populations, for example. By the same token, if it is truly impossible to estimate future dynamics, a naive technique is the only possible choice.

Whenever reasonable guesses or confident forecasts of future dynamics are possible, it makes more sense to look at causal techniques, even in the short run. The choice is always a matter of judgment, of course, as to what is sufficiently reasonable or confident, but naive forecasting techniques are inherently riskier in most cases. Depending on the technique, naive forecasting can lead to estimates of enormous changes in utilization, especially where small numbers are involved, yet incorporate no reason for such changes. In a situation of absolute ignorance it is almost always wisest to assume no change in utilization rather than forecast a major change with no basis for explanation.

*Causal* techniques rely on the relationship between utilization of health services and another factor. They treat future health services utilization as a function of what will happen to some other factors or of what has happened already. By definition, causal techniques require that information on at least one other factor be examined as a basis for forecasting health services utilization. They assume that there is some stable, quantitative relationship between health services utilization and the other factors. It is not necessary that this relationship be truly causal, despite the name, as long as it is identifiable and persistent.

Adding in another factor obviously complicates the task of forecasting as compared to most naive techniques. On the other hand it recognizes that there are factors that either affect or are strongly associated with health services utilization and that can be useful in estimating future utilization. In order to forecast utilization as the function of some other factors, it is usually necessary to have a confident and precise estimate of the factors. Hence causal techniques introduce the possibility of using arbitrary or unreasoned estimates of the future of one factor in order to produce a supposedly objective and reasonable estimate of future utilization.

This possibility can be avoided in two ways. First, some factors, e.g., population, might be subject to such precise, confident, and usually accurate forecasting that they constitute reasonable bases for predicting health services utilization. If so, and if the *relationship* between the factor and utilization is stable, good forecasts can result. Second, if a time-lagging approach is used, present, hence *measurable*, data on related factors can be used to predict utilization as long as the time-lagged or delayed relationship is stable. As long as the relationships between causal factors and health services utilization can be identified and either are stable or change predictably, causal forecasting techniques will tend to produce better results than naive alternatives.

A major advantage of causal techniques is that they can be used for intermediate and long-range forecasting, as well as short-range. For this use, intermediate and long-range forecasts of the causal factors are required, but if precise and confident forecasts of the factors are available, using the technique is no more complicated to look farther into the future than to look at the short range. Because precision and confidence tend to diminish over time, of course, the precision and confidence of causally forecast utilization must also diminish.

## Passive versus Intervention

One of the most important choices relative to forecasting health services utilization is between an interventionist and passive approach to the task. For a health care organization forecasting its own utilization, a totally passive approach is unlikely to be the only choice. There are times, however, in the short run when a passive approach is the only logical alternative if no possible steps can take enough effect quickly. On the other hand a passive forecast may be made first just to see if any intervention is called for. If a confident, precise estimate of future utilization matches or exceeds expectations or requirements, there may be no need to consider interventions, hence no need for an interventionist forecasting technique.

Interventionist forecasts may routinely be made and compared to passive results merely to consider the advisability of intervention. If the cost of the intervention is greater than the value of the difference in expected utilization or if there is really no significant difference, the intervention would be downgraded. The relative precision and confidence of the passive versus interventionist forecast determine whether valid choices can be made.

For some organizations passive forecasts may be the only choice. They may lack mechanisms for influencing future utilization, not know of any effective methods, or be reluctant to use any that they know. It has been common for publicly funded organizations to rely on passive forecasting lest they be accused of manipulating public behavior. Health care organizations in general have only recently recognized the potential of marketing concepts and techniques for influencing utilization.

Naive forecasting techniques are always passive because they foresee nothing changing. This represents another reason to avoid naive techniques for anything but the short run; they permit no intervention. Causal techniques on the other hand may be used in either passive or interventionist modes. The key is whether the causal factors are subject to influence, i.e., whether influenceable factors are incorporated in the technique. Forecasts for which utilization is a function of population size or demographic factors would rarely be open to intervention, although those based on psychographic or health system factors would (see Chapter 8).

## DATA REQUIREMENTS

For most forecasting situations the availability of data has a significant effect on what techniques are possible and promising. Naive techniques by definition rely on the availability of sufficient past utilization data to form the basis for extrapolating to the future. Causal techniques by definition require sufficient understanding of the dynamics affecting utilization and at least accurate data on present utilization in order to work. Whether sufficient appropriate data are available first determines what forecasting techniques can be used. The quality of such data then greatly influences how accurate and precise forecasts can be.

Past and present utilization data plus information on causal factors linked to such utilization must be as precise and accurate as possible in order for forecasts based on them to be at all precise and accurate. Any imprecision in data tends to be magnified into greater imprecision in forecasts based on those data. Any inaccuracy in data may completely destroy the potential for accuracy in forecasting.

If the decisions to be made on the basis of forecasts of utilization are at all important, hence making the choice of forecasting technique critical, then the precision and accuracy of data are worthy of substantial attention. Data supplied by others (secondary data) should be checked against other sources, with any analyses (sums, products, etc.) recalculated. If hospital admissions, length of stay, and patient days are reported, for example, they should be checked to ensure that admissions times length of stay equals patient days. Data should always be treated as potentially containing error, with checking and double-checking worth the effort.

The quantity and type of data available greatly influence the sorts of forecasting techniques that can be considered. Substantial data on past utilization should be available if any sort of extrapolation technique is to be considered. These data should be available for exactly the same services or exactly the same pattern to be forecast. If reports of past utilization do not specify the service category or patient characteristics that must be forecast for a given decision, then only two choices are available. Either the organization's own records must be examined to improve the data, or some other forecasting technique must be used.

In general it is usually a wise move to maintain utilization data in as comprehensive and integrated a fashion as possible. Merging patient medical record data and operating cost data with billing and collections data, for example, is necessary to forecasting the profitability implications of future utilization. Merging diagnostic, treatment, and service cost information is key to forecasting the consequences of specific utilization patterns under DRG payment. If data bases can at least be keyed to the same base, e.g., a patient identification number, combined analyses are possible even if the data systems are not actually merged.

Having a comprehensive, integrated data base facilitates the development of data required in forecasting and greatly extends the range of possible choices. In designing a data system it is wise to consider forecasting applications together with financial, management, reporting, and other requirements. It is always easier to use data that were recorded and stored appropriately in the first place than it is to reconstitute data in order to employ a desired forecasting technique. With the available types of mainframe and microprocessor computers, comprehensive, integrated data bases are easy to develop and maintain and are well worth the effort.

## SUMMARY

Choices required in the forecasting of utilization involve time frames over which use is to be forecast, the determination as to whether a naive or causal technique is preferred, and the choice between a passive or an interventionist approach. The time frame selection addresses the period over which use is to be forecast: its beginning, duration, and end. The period selection is a function of the lead time required before the decision to be made will take effect and the length of time that decision, when coupled with utilization, will affect operating performance. Specific note should be made of when and how corrections can be made in the decision if revisions are called for in the utilization forecast.

Naive forecasting techniques are based on a rational decision that nothing useful is known about the reasons for past utilization levels. Only the levels themselves, the past history of the use of a given health service, are felt to be the proper basis for forecasting its future. Causal techniques insist that the past and future of at least one other reality should be considered when forecasting utilization. The identification of that reality and the determination of its relationship to utilization levels become the basis for forecasts.

If a causal technique is chosen, the forecaster has the option of dealing with causal factors that can or cannot be influenced. If such factors cannot be modified by the organization, the only choice is to take a passive approach to forecasting. If one or more factors can be influenced, the organization may choose an interventionist approach, assuming that it is willing to make the effort necessary to bring about a desired utilization level.

Accurate and precise data on past and present utilization greatly increase the range of available forecasting options and the precision and accuracy of any forecasts based on them. Data to be used in forecasting should be carefully checked, recalculated where possible, and externally validated. Data systems designed and maintained by each provider should be suited to forecasting as well as other planning, management, and reporting purposes. Any forecast based on data can only be as good as the data.

# Chapter 3

# Evaluating Techniques

With a wide variety of available forecasting techniques from which to choose, selecting the most appropriate techniques is anything but a routine matter. The choices made regarding what is to be forecast, over which periods of time, and those made between naive versus causal and passive versus interventionist approaches greatly narrow the range. The rest of the job should be based on careful, systematic evaluation. The inherent assumptions of each technique, whether implicit or explicit, should be identified and examined. Where possible, the techniques should be tested before final selection is made or the final forecast accepted as the basis for making a decision.

The value of any forecasting technique compared to any other should be assessed relative to the decisions that will be made based on the forecast. With this in mind, there are likely to be three critical considerations relative to the process of forecasting and three more relative to the output. Process considerations include the cost of using a technique, the relative complexity and difficulty of using it, and its ability to produce the needed forecast in time for decision making. Output considerations relate to the precision of data, the confidence of the forecaster that it will be accurate, and the acceptability of the forecast to those who should accept it.

## PROCESS CONSIDERATIONS

*Cost* considerations include cost of the data required for the technique, cost of any software and hardware used in processing the data, plus the time and effort of personnel involved. Data requirements for some naive techniques can be virtually nil, although for others, such as Box-Jenkins and ARIMA, they can be substantial. Data required for causal techniques, especially those based on multiple causal factors (see Chapter 11) may have to be purchased from outside sources or collected on an original basis. If causal factors must be forecast, the costs of those forecasts are added to the cost of forecasting utilization. If consultants or other outside experts are to be used in collecting data, costs can become considerable.

The *process* of analyzing the data can add substantial amounts to the cost of forecasting. Increasingly software packages designed for forecasting are becoming available for microcomputers, enabling complex techniques to be employed by desk-top computers. Even pocket calculators can be programmed to perform sophisticated calculations for use in forecasting. On the other hand growing sophistication regarding the available techniques tends to move us away from the simple, low-cost techniques. Some firms specialize in specific forecasting techniques for which they charge rather handsomely. It must always be remembered, of course, that the complexity and cost of the forecasting technique do not guarantee its value. Poor data or assumptions destroy the value of the best software and hardware while retaining their costs.

*Time and effort* of the organization's own employees represent another cost, though one less likely to be as clearly identified or as carefully considered. There are advantages to using one's own employees in any forecasting effort likely to be repeated. Once they learn the technique, they can employ it, probably with much less trouble and potentially greater skill, the next time the forecast must be made. If consultants are used, the organization may become dependent on them every time the same forecast must be made. This may be good for the outsiders but expensive for the organization. Other considerations may limit the extent to which insiders can and should be used.

*Complexity and difficulty* of the forecasting technique determine whether it is within the capability of the organization to use, how much it costs to use it, and the time needed to employ it. They can also affect the extent to which the forecaster has confidence in the forecast if the technique has many places where errors might occur. Moreover techniques that are complicated and difficult to use are likely to present quite a challenge to describe to those who must accept their validity. Unless such people are likely to be impressed by sophisticated techniques that they don't understand, difficulties in describing and explaining a technique may result in difficulties in getting the forecast accepted.

*Timeliness* of forecasting is an obvious but important consideration. The timing of the decision dictates when the forecast must be available. A short time may mean that only simple techniques can be considered even though more sophisticated alternatives might be preferred. A long time should not lead to automatic preference of a sophisticated technique unless the more sophisticated truly promises better output. By the same token the most sophisticated technique with precise, confident, and highly acceptable output would be wasted if it can't produce a forecast when needed.

## OUTPUT CONSIDERATIONS

Precision of forecasts is a critical consideration in decision making. Unfortunately no general guide or standard applies to forecasts, even for specific time frames. The precision needed of any forecast is a function of the decision and its sensitivity to the range of utilization levels entailed in the forecast. If utilization must be at least 15,000 visits for a given decision to be made, a forecast that is 20,000 plus or minus 5,000 is terribly imprecise but all that is needed to make the decision. If the output were 15,000 plus or minus 1,000, the forecast might be useless, even though quite precise. Only the decision context can say whether a forecast is precise enough, but techniques that tend to produce precise forecasts are generally more valuable.

*Confidence* in the likely accuracy of a forecast is probably the most important consideration regardless of its precision. Confidence, unlike any of the process considerations or precision, cannot be quantified well. The forecaster may be able to subjectively assign confidence ratings, e.g., 0 percent to 100 percent confidence, as a way of judging alternative techniques, but such subjective numbers have no other use. Confidence is likely to be related inversely to precision because it is easier to have confidence that future utilization will be within some large range than that it will be right near some specific point estimate.

Confidence can be affected by the quantity and quality of data used in the forecasting technique. It is also affected by the extent to which the technique is understood by the forecaster, hence by its complexity and sophistication. Confidence should be influenced by the type of assumptions inherent in the technique employed, which is why they should be identified and examined. The time frame for the forecast also affects confidence because the farther in the future we look, the less confidence we can have in the forecast.

Reasoned confidence in a forecast should be based on a good understanding of the dynamics affecting utilization of health services. If a naive forecasting technique is used, the forecaster should be convinced that those dynamics are persistent and will not change in the time frame of the forecast. Naive techniques may be used because no understanding of the dynamics exists, but then confidence will be lacking. If a causal technique is used, the forecaster should be convinced that the relationships incorporated in the technique will persist or change predictably over the time frame of the forecast and that measures or forecasts of related factors used to predict utilization are valid.

*Acceptability* of forecasts is important whenever the decisions based on them are made by or subject to approval by anyone other than the forecaster. Whether others have the same confidence in a forecast as the forecaster is affected by the quantity and quality of data used, the forecasting techniques employed, and the extent to which the forecast fits preconceptions and biases of those who review it. Each of these factors should be considered by the forecaster in developing an estimate of future utilization. The best forecast from a technical point of view is wasted if it is not believed and accepted in the decision-making and ratification proc ess.

Data can influence acceptance through its quantity and quality. The use of little data, or few people in subjective estimates, tends to look unscientific even if it may be justified. The more important the decision, and the forecast to it, and the more people who must ratify the decision, the more importance the quantity of data used is likely to have. Quality of data is equally important. A measurement or estimate of the past or present that is not accepted by decision makers or reviewers leads to rejection of the forecast and the decision. Population forecasts that seem biased or unlikely have the same effect. Quantity and quality of data must be carefully balanced to ensure what will seem to be an adequate data base but not result in rejection of any of its components. The use of external, objective sources of data is generally superior in this regard to developing the data base internally, unless the organization's own records are adequate.

The forecasting technique should be sophisticated enough to be impressive or state-of-the-art, and also capable of being described and explained by the forecaster. Unless the technique or the forecaster has a reputation that eliminates all doubt, those who must accept the forecast tend to doubt a technique that they don't understand even if they don't express that overtly. Careful explanation of the technique may be necessary, including illustration of how specific data were employed to produce specific forecasts. The forecaster must prepare illustrative and explanatory material for such a use.

In almost all cases where forecasts are used to make decisions people involved have preconceived notions about the future and preferences regarding the proper decision. Where the forecast disagrees with their own notions or the decision violates their prejudice, conflicts are likely. Unless the forecast is so clearly unchallengeable and the decision follows so inexorably from it as to override doubt, it is wise to address preconceptions and prejudices early in the decision process. Where the acceptance of a decision is as important as its being correct, and is open to doubt, the participation of those who must accept it in developing the forecast is likely to be useful.

Such political input into forecasting is also capable of increasing the technical validity of the forecast. Individuals with preconceived notions may have insights into the dynamics affecting utilization that are new to the forecaster. Conflict theory explains that involving people with different preferences in making a decision increases the quantity and quality of information considered, even though it may make reaching a decision more difficult and time-consuming. If acceptance is critical and conflict potential high, the process is likely to work better if those who must make and ratify a decision based on a forecast are involved at the forecast stage. If they can participate in developing a forecast that they accept, they are much more likely to go along with the decision based on it.

This is especially true if an interventionist approach to forecasting is used. Those who are part of or approve the interventions needed to achieve a forecast level of utilization are more likely to go along if they participate in making the forecast. Physicians who must alter their behavior in order to reach an intervention-based level of outpatient surgery volume are much more likely to do so if they developed the forecast used in making a decision to create or expand such a program, for example.

## ASSUMPTIONS

One of the most useful rules of systematic thinking calls for identifying and objectively examining all assumptions used in reaching conclusions. This is especially true in forecasting because any estimate of the future is necessarily a leap of faith into the unknown. Many of the assumptions essential to a forecasting technique are likely to be unstated, hence not open to examination on the surface. The duty of the forecaster is to identify such assumptions clearly, both when employing the technique and when presenting the forecast for consideration. If there are any serious doubts about the assumptions intrinsic to a technique, there should be limited confidence in the forecast that results.

Naive forecasts by definition assume that past patterns of utilization will persist unchanged into the future. Use of the past 5 weeks' utilization to project the next 5, for example, assumes that we are in the middle of a 10-week period of stable dynamics whose first half is inexorably related to its second. A devil's advocate or Murphy's law review of such an assumption is likely to be useful. The advocate looks for alternative assumptions that might be equally valid or even more likely than those in the technique. The Murphy's approach looks for all factors that could go wrong, i.e., could cause the assumptions to be invalid.

Causal forecasts assume that the relationships that they employ are stable or will change predictably and that no other factors not incorporated in the causal model will affect future utilization to a significant degree. These assumptions deserve explicit examination just as much as those inherent in naive techniques. The use of a devil's advocate or Murphy's law review is equally appropriate here. Specific application of these assumption-testing approaches relative to individual forecasting techniques and applications are discussed in subsequent chapters. They should be routinely employed by the forecaster in developing and presenting forecasts.

The best way to think of forecasting assumptions is in the context of change dynamics. Given the factors that affect utilization of health services, what changes in these factors produced observable changes in utilization behavior? How will these factors change in the future, and what impact will such changes have on utilization behavior? Even if the forecasting technique being employed is a naive one, the review of assumptions should always be causal. Utilization of health services is clearly related to characteristics of the users of services, the providers of services, and the environment in which both interact. The extent to which changes in these characteristics are likely and foreseeable is basic to the forecasting process. Only where changes are unlikely or impossible to foresee should they be omitted from a forecast.

It is particularly important that the assumptions intrinsic to a forecasting technique be identified and justified to decision makers and ratifiers as part of the forecast presented. Not to do so is essentially dishonest and unprofessional of the forecaster. Moreover getting additional insights into the validity of assumptions is likely to be useful from a technical as well as political perspective. Finally, having others discuss and approve or modify the assumptions, hence the forecast itself, protects the forecaster from getting all the blame if the forecast is significantly in error. All that any forecaster can and should promise is to use the best data, technique, and assumptions available. If they were used and the future moves in unexpected ways, that is merely the nature of the future. If assumptions used in the technique were questionable but were not questioned or even identified by the forecaster, then negative repercussions are both likely and deserved.

## TESTING OF TECHNIQUES

In addition to identifying and testing the assumptions intrinsic to a given forecasting technique, the technique itself should be tested wherever feasible. Such testing in most cases involves applying the technique entirely to past data. Such testing against past data does not *prove* that it will work in the future. On the other hand, if a technique doesn't work on past data, the forecaster has a strong basis for questioning whether it is likely to work in the future. The testing of techniques is a useful device for screening out techniques at least. In conjunction with choices regarding time frames, naive versus causal and passive versus interventionist techniques, screening for past performance should leave the forecaster with only a few realistic choices to consider among the vast number of forecasting techniques.

If a naive projection technique is to be used (see Part II), additional past data should be gathered for use in testing the technique if such data are available. If utilization data from five recent periods are to be used to project the next one or two periods, then utilization data from past sets of five periods should be examined to see how well they projected the one or two periods following each set. If the mean and standard deviation of the errors produced by testing the technique are minimal, then a better notion of its likely precision in the future is possible. If past errors have been significant, the forecaster should at least ask why errors should be less in the future.

Testing causal techniques on past data may be a little more complicated but is equally worthwhile. If a simple or multiple correlation technique is to be used based on the past 10 years to predict the next 5, then data from the prior 10 years can be looked at to see if the correlations hold for the first 5 years of the past 10 (see Part III). If correlation coefficients were different in prior past years, the forecaster should at least question why they should be expected to be the same in the future.

In a classic article published over fifteen years ago, Paul Feldstein and Jeremiah German compared three alternative models for predicting hospital utilization behavior by populations. They tested these models by means of splitting a prior period (1952–1961) into two halves, then using data on the first half to predict the second. They indicated that the selection of a 10-year period was based on a convention espoused by the Joint Committee of the American Hospital Association and the U.S. Public Health Service, Division of Hospital Facilities, in their 1961 report. This report recommended using as many years of past data as the years to be covered by a forecast. Thus, to predict five years ahead, five years of past data are required. Such a convention is still in common use.

The results of the Feldstein and German analysis indicated that when forecasting statewide population use rates (patient days per thousand population per year), a least-squares linear regression based on past data worked well. It worked better in fact than predictions based on bed supplies or those based on multiple regressions using econometric variables.

The authors warned, however, that linear extrapolations of past data work only when underlying factors causing past changes in behavior continue to change and impact on behavior in a consistent fashion. They also warned that highly aggregated data such as the statewide use rates that they employed are likely to be better subjects for trend forecasting than less aggregated data such as utilization rates for small communities.

In an effort to update these results and to assess the values and risks of trend forecasting, analyses were conducted of population use rates for populations smaller and larger than those of U.S. states. The small populations chosen for analysis were residents of the 42 counties in Idaho, whose utilization behavior was analyzed for the period of 1968–1977. These counties were also aggregated into seven multicounty regions for a second order of analysis. Statewide trends in utilization were also identified for comparison purposes.

The large populations were residents of four regions of the United States commonly used for analysis by the National Center for Health Statistics. Utilization behavior of the residents of the Northeast, North Central, South, and West regions was analyzed over the period of 1970–1979. Such behavior was examined on an age-specific basis, with utilization reported for the cohorts 0 to 14, 15 to 44, 45 to 64, and 65-plus years of age. A higher level of aggregation was achieved by examining utilization behavior by region across all ages and by age cohort across all regions, as well as by examining utilization behavior by the entire U.S. population.

In both samples hospital utilization behavior was broken down into three measures: annual admissions per thousand population (admission rate); average number of days in hospital per admission (average length of stay); and annual patient days per thousand population, the product of the first two (use rate). In forecasting it is common practice to break down use rates into their two components, then combine the two to forecast use rates, though many practitioners forecast use rates alone.

## TREND ANALYSIS

The trends in annual utilization were calculated for the first five years in both samples. Although individual cases followed a variety of idiosyncratic curvilinear trends, the best trend form for all cases taken as a whole proved to be a simple linear time series regression of the form

$$y = a + bx$$

where $y$ = utilization in any given year

$a$ = a constant
$b$ = a coefficient
$x$ = the order of the year in a time series sequence ($x$ = 1 through 5 were used in calculating the trend values for $a$ and $b$)

As shown in Table 3-1, a simple linear regression described the typical five-year period with admirable though imperfect accuracy. Median $r^2$ values for the various utilization measures ranged from a low of .314 to a high of .802. Half of the cases produced $r^2$ values in excess of .500, in which the trend accounted for at least half the year-to-year changes in utilization behavior. These results suggest that linear trends did at least a fair job of characterizing the first five years of the test periods.

**Directional Accuracy**

The first trend value checked against the subsequent five-year period was the sign of the coefficient or slope of the trend line forecast. The sign of the first five years was compared to the sign of the second (the negative sign indicates decreasing utilization; positive, increasing). As indicated in Table 3-2, results for individual county populations in Idaho were disappointing. The first-half trend correctly predicted the second in only 31.0 percent of the cases for admission rates, 47.6 percent for length of stay,

**Table 3-1** Trend Strength in First Five Years' Utilization Measures

| Population Studied | Utilization Measure | Median $r^2$ for Trends |
|---|---|---|
| Idaho counties $n$ = 42 | Admission rate (AR) | .524 |
| | Length of stay (LOS) | .416 |
| | Use rate (UR) | .603 |
| Idaho regions $n$ = 8 | Admission rate (AR) | .607 |
| | Length of stay (LOS) | .448 |
| | Use rate (UR) | .487 |
| United States regional age cohorts $n$ = 16 | Admission rate (AR) | .510 |
| | Length of stay (LOS) | .802 |
| | Use rate (UR) | .370 |
| United States combined populations $n$ = 9 | Admission rate (AR) | .524 |
| | Length of stay (LOS) | .418 |
| | Use rate (UR) | .314 |

**Table 3-2** Directional Accuracy of Five-Year Trend

| Population | Utilization Measure | Number of Cases | Number Correct | Percentage Correct |
|---|---|---|---|---|
| Idaho counties | AR | 42 | 13 | 31.0 |
| | LOS | 42 | 20 | 47.6 |
| | UR | 42 | 23 | 54.8 |
| Total | | 126 | 56 | 44.4 |
| Idaho region | AR | 8 | 2 | 25.0 |
| | LOS | 8 | 7 | 87.5 |
| | UR | 8 | 3 | 37.5 |
| Total | | 24 | 12 | 50.0 |
| United States | AR | 16 | 10 | 62.5 |
| regional | LOS | 16 | 15 | 93.8 |
| age cohorts | UR | 16 | 13 | 81.3 |
| Total | | 48 | 38 | 79.2 |
| United States | AR | 9 | 8 | 88.9 |
| combined | LOS | 9 | 7 | 77.8 |
| | UR | 9 | 3 | 33.3 |
| Total | | 27 | 18 | 66.7 |

and 54.8 percent for use rates. For all three measures the trend accurately predicted change direction less than half the time.

Accuracy improved somewhat when populations were aggregated into regions. Although admission rate trends were correct in only two of eight cases, and use rate trends three of eight, trends were correct in seven of eight cases for length of stay. Where overall accuracy for counties was only 56 of 126, or 44.4 percent, the trends correctly predicted direction of changes in utilization behavior in 12 of 24 cases for regional populations (50.0 percent). Because flipping a coin should yield 50 percent accuracy, however, neither of these represents good performance.

With larger populations, directional accuracy of the trend forecasts improves. For regional age cohorts the first five years correctly predicted the directional trend of the second in 62.5 percent of the cases for admission rates, 93.8 percent for length of stay, and 81.3 percent for use rates. Overall the trends were correct in 38 of 48 cases, or 79.2 percent. Aggregating populations still further did not significantly improve trend accuracy. For national age cohorts, separate regions, and the United States as a whole, accuracy diminished dramatically to 66.7 percent overall.

**Comparative Accuracy**

More than the direction of future change, past trends should give us a good estimate of future values for admission rates, length of stay, and use rates. To determine how accurate the first five-year trends were, their forecasts of tenth-year values for each of the utilization behavior measures were compared to the actual measures for the tenth year. A percentage error was determined by dividing the predicted value by the actual measure.

For comparison, alternative forecasts were also developed from the same five years' data. One alternative was the mean value for the first five years' measures. The second alternative was the fifth, i.e., last, year in the period used to calculate the trend. These alternatives represent the more conservative assumption that no trend was present at all or that if present in the past, would not continue.

As shown in Table 3-3, the accuracy of past trends in predicting specific values for future utilization was disappointing. For individual Idaho counties mean error percentages ranged from 29.2 percent to 39.5 percent over the three utilization measures. The five-year mean was a far better predictor on average for all three measures. The fifth-year values proved the best predictors by far for all three, with error percentages from one-half to one-third those associated with the trend forecasts. Whether errors averaging 11.5 percent to 13.4 percent would represent acceptable performance is another question, but errors of 30 percent to 40 percent would surely not.

---

**Table 3-3** Comparative Accuracy Forecast versus Actual Tenth Year

| Population | Utilization Measure | Five-Year Trend | Mean Percentage Errors Five-Year Mean | Fifth Year |
|---|---|---|---|---|
| Idaho counties | AR | 37.2 | 19.8 | 13.4 |
| $n = 42$ | LOS | 29.2 | 16.0 | 12.6 |
| | UR | 39.5 | 21.2 | 11.5 |
| Mean | | 35.3 | 19.0 | 12.5 |
| Idaho regions | AR | 13.7 | 9.8 | 7.4 |
| $n = 8$ | LOS | 7.9 | 12.0 | 10.5 |
| | UR | 21.5 | 15.0 | 14.5 |
| Mean | | 14.4 | 12.3 | 10.8 |
| United States | AR | 8.3 | 8.2 | 5.6 |
| regional | LOS | 10.1 | 11.7 | 8.0 |
| age cohorts | UR | 8.9 | 6.7 | 5.6 |
| $n = 16$ | | | | |
| Mean | | 9.1 | 8.9 | 6.4 |
| United States | AR | 3.8 | 10.2 | 6.0 |
| combined | LOS | 8.0 | 10.1 | 7.1 |
| $n = 9$ | UR | 8.2 | 3.8 | 2.9 |
| Mean | | 6.7 | 8.0 | 5.3 |

At the next level of aggregation, examining trend forecasting accuracy for the multicounty regions in Idaho yielded somewhat better results. Regionwide length-of-stay values were predicted with a median error of only 7.9 percent, though admission rates averaged 13.7 percent error and use rates, 21.5 percent. Still the trend forecasts compete more favorably with the five-year mean and fifth-year alternatives where they had been distinctly inferior for individual county population utilization behavior.

For the U.S. regional age cohorts, the five-year trend forecasts were somewhat more accurate in predicting utilization behavior, with median error rates ranging from 8.3 to 10.1 over the three measures. Even for this level of aggregation, however, the trend forecasts were on the whole less accurate than the forecasts based on the average of the first five years and distinctly less accurate than the forecasts based on the fifth year. At the highest level of aggregation—national age cohorts, regions, and the U.S. population as a whole—forecasting errors dropped only slightly. For the first time the trend forecasting errors were on average less than those from using the five-year average but still worse than the errors from using the fifth year as a constant value.

Across both samples, at all levels of aggregation, forecasting errors resulting from trend extrapolation were greater than those based on assuming no change in utilization behavior. Although the errors produced by both trend and no-change forecasting diminished as aggregation levels increased, the superiority of the no-change forecast continued at all levels.

**Trend Strength and Forecasting Accuracy**

It is generally believed that the stronger a trend is, the more useful and reliable it should be in forecasting. To test this belief, the coefficient of determination or $r^2$ value for each five-year trend was compared to its accuracy. Correlation measures were made of the relationship between $r^2$ value and error percentage for each trend across all three utilization measures in each sample.

As shown in Table 3-4, the strength of the five-year trend, measured in terms of $r^2$ value, was not at all associated with better forecasting accuracy. The product-moment correlations between trend strength and error percentage were low and not statistically significant. In only 5 of the 12 cases was the sign of the correlation even in the predicted direction (negative). For the other cases higher $r^2$ values were slightly associated with higher errors. In terms of ability to explain errors, trend strength explained at most a small proportion of the forecasting errors.

The $r^2$ values that measure the strength of the past trend reflect merely how well the trend accounts for past changes. Based on this analysis such

**Table 3-4** Correlation of Five-Year Trend Strength with Trend-Forecasting Accuracy

| Population | Utilization Measure | Correlation: Trend $r^2$ with Percentage Error | Coefficient of Determination |
|---|---|---|---|
| Idaho counties | AR | −.051 | .003 |
| $n = 42$ | LOS | −.028 | .001 |
| | UR | .118 | .014 |
| Idaho regions | AR | −.436 | .190 |
| $n = 8$ | LOS | .134 | .018 |
| | UR | .039 | .002 |
| United States regional age cohorts $n = 16$ | AR | .322 | .104 |
| | LOS | −.111 | .012 |
| | UR | .225 | .051 |
| United States combined $n = 9$ | AR | .072 | .005 |
| | LOS | −.606 | .367 |
| | UR | .372 | .138 |

strength has no particular association with the probability that the trend will persevere. Because the forecasting accuracy of trends is based on their perseverance, there is no particular reason why the strength of past trends should be associated with perseverance. The strength of past trends reflects the past but doesn't say anything about the future.

### Discussion

These findings should come as no particular surprise. Past trends characterize the past with varying degrees of accuracy. There is no intrinsic necessity that such trends characterize the future as well. Traditional trend-adjusting techniques such as exponential smoothing are designed to give greater weight to more recent experience. Moreover trend forecasting techniques are generally used to predict only one year ahead, assuming minimal perseverance.

When faced with the necessity of forecasting utilization behavior of populations a number of years from now, it is necessary to understand what causes change rather than assume the perseverance of past change patterns. During the 1960s hospital utilization was presumably affected by the Medicare and Medicaid legislation and its stimulation of demand by reducing financial barriers. During the 1970s such utilization was influenced more by attempts to control it via utilization review. Through both decades changes in the age structures of population, medical technology, alternatives to inpatient care, and physician attitudes toward hospitalization had some effect.

To predict the future beyond the next year, especially to anticipate utilization behavior 5 to 10 years ahead, we should probably deal with the dynamics affecting such behavior to the best of our understanding. There is no reason that past trends should automatically persevere, and analysis of the recent past indicates that they don't persevere in a reliable fashion. If we truly don't understand or can't predict the dynamics of change, a forecast of no change appears to be the safer assumption.

A trend extrapolation forecast of the form tested makes a risky, albeit unstated, assumption. That is, the phenomenon to be forecast is in the midst of a long-term linear trend whose first half is an exact copy of the second. To forecast the next 5 years based on the past 5 using a linear extrapolation, we must assume that we are in the midst of a 10-year linear trend with perfect symmetry. Such an assumption is by no means the best or safest assumption to make. The kinds of errors that resulted from trend extrapolation applied to county and even multicounty populations were uncomfortably great. Even for larger populations they were greater than a steady-state assumption.

It can only be hoped that by putting our minds to analyzing the dynamics of change and estimating the impacts of foreseeable developments in factors that affect hospital utilization, we can improve on any simple mathematical approach. Such approaches may appear objective and even scientific but, when based entirely on past data, are likely to be extremely unreliable forecasters.

## SUMMARY

With the decision-making context established and a wide variety of forecasting techniques available, choices must be made. Such choices should involve consideration of the process used in forecasting and the outputs of that process. Process considerations include the financial costs, logistical complexity, and timeliness with which a given technique can be employed. Output considerations cover the precision of utilization levels forecast, the level of confidence that can be reasonably placed in such a forecast, and the degree to which the technique employed can be explained to and accepted by whoever will make and ratify the decisions based on the forecast.

The selection of a forecasting technique should include specific attention to the assumptions implicit in each technique. These assumptions are rarely made explicit but represent necessary underpinnings for each approach being considered. If the basic underlying assumptions cannot be reasonably accepted, then the technique shouldn't be employed.

Wherever possible a proposed technique should be tested by trying it out on past situations. If the technique would have worked given the information available at some past time in forecasting the present, it might well, but not necessarily, work again. If it would have failed in the past, serious questions ought to be raised regarding its likelihood of working in the future.

---

**Annotated Bibliography**

**Bell, D.** "Twelve Modes of Prediction—A Preliminary Sorting." *Daedalus* 93 (Summer 1964): 845.
Discusses a wide variety of forecasting techniques with emphasis on long-range forecasting.

**Berki, S.** "Demand and Utilization." Chapter 6 in *Hospital Economics.* Lexington, Mass: D. C. Heath, 1972, p. 121.
Reviews the literature on forecasting utilization of hospital services.

**Cantor, J.** *Pragmatic Forecasting.* New York: American Management Association, 1971.
Discusses the selection of forecasting technique based on the range of time involved and precision required in making the decision.

**Chambers, J., et al.** "How to Choose the Right Forecasting Technique." *Harvard Business Review* 49, no. 4 (July–August 1971): 45.
Discusses how to select a forecasting technique based on its application in decision making.

**Fildes, R.** "Quantitative Forecasting—The State of the Art: Extrapolative Models." *Journal of the Operations Research Society* 30, no. 8 (August 1979): 691.
Discusses alternative extrapolation techniques and their application with evidence on their accuracy in practice.

**Golden, C., et al.** "Good Forecasting Builds Good Budgets." *Hospital Financial Management,* (August 1981): p. 18.
Compares accuracy of Box-Jenkins, modified exponential smoothing and percentage change forecasts; finds Box-Jenkins best, percentage change worst.

**Harrington, M.** "Forecasting Areawide Demand for Health Services: A Critical Review of Major Techniques and Their Application." *Inquiry* 14, no. 3 (September 1977): 254.
Discusses six categories of forecasting techniques, their strengths, and limitations applied to areawide utilization levels.

**Jones, M.** *Technology Assessment Methodology: Some Basic Propositions.* Washington, D.C.: Mitre Corporation, 1971.
Provides descriptions of forecasting techniques and problems in applications.

**Martino, J.** "Technological Forecasting—An Overview." *Management Science* 26, no. 1 (January 1980): 28.
Discusses the range of forecasting techniques available, with special emphasis on recent developments and use of techniques.

# Part II

# Projection Techniques

By definition a projection forecasting technique relies on identifying a pattern in past utilization of health services. This pattern can be assessed to see how closely it reflects observed utilization. If the pattern seems to fit observations well, a leap of faith is made and the pattern is *projected* into the future. Such a projection can be accomplished by drawing straight or curved lines or by using quantitative expressions. Closeness of fit between observed utilization and the projection pattern can likewise be assessed either visually or mathematically.

All projection forecasting techniques are naive in that they employ only information on past utilization to project future utilization. Projection techniques treat future utilization levels as functions of their own history rather than as functions of any other factors. Essentially projections rely on the principle of analogy, the idea that what has happened is the best clue to what will happen. A projection assumes that the future will be just like the past or that the past is part of a longer-range pattern, which can be identified from its early development.

The beauty of projection techniques lies in their simplicity. They may appear objective in that past utilization data are used rather than subjective conjecture to forecast the future. The decision to employ a projection technique rather than some other approach is purely subjective, however. Moreover selection of what pattern to rely on, even of what period of time to use to establish the pattern, is a subjective judgment. Every projection chooses to believe that the future will replicate the past. The reasonableness of this belief ought to be established before the projection is accepted as the best or even a reasonable estimate of future utilization.

The issue of time is a critical one in projection forecasting. Some minimum time is required in order to identify a pattern in past utilization at all. A minimum of five past periods is usually recommended. Whether to employ more than five periods of past data is a significant issue. Looking backward through more than five periods can alter the pattern and modify the assessment of fit between observations and the projection model. It can result in preference for an entirely different model, e.g., a curvilinear rather than a linear projection. Extending observations farther into the past could lead to identification of a cyclical pattern rather than a trend or suggest that no time trend is present where one might have appeared to be in recent data.

There is no way to decide how many periods of past data to use except through human judgment. The best number is whatever is sufficient to identify a pattern that will persist. It is the persistence of a pattern, not its fit with past data, that makes it a good forecasting tool. A measurement of fit, whether visual or mathematical, merely shows how well a pattern describes the past. A perfect fit is no more likely to be replicated in the future than a less-than-perfect fit, especially if the factors affecting utilization behave differently in the future than in the past.

The goodness of fit between past utilization data and one of the projection patterns being considered for use is typically the basis for selecting which pattern to use. Selecting a model based on the visual or mathematical proximity between it and observed utilization in the past seems reasonable enough. A pattern that accurately describes the past is more likely to project the future accurately than one that is less accurate, *assuming that all causal factors behave as they did*. Some measures of fit, however, favor patterns of extreme change (see Chapter 4). Because continual extreme change is a rare phenomenon indeed, there is danger in relying on past fit alone. Where the best fit pattern is one of rapid change, forecasters should be even more wary of assuming the pattern's persistence, especially far into the future.

A choice always inherent in a projection technique is how far into the future to project. The answer to this question requires exactly the same sort of judgment as needed to decide how many past periods of data to use in identifying a pattern. The best answer requires knowing how far into the future the past patterns can confidently be expected to persist. The better the dynamics producing past patterns are understood, the better a judgment can be made. In the absence of confident understanding of change dynamics and confident expectation that past patterns will persist, the best guess is one of no change. In the absence of such confidence, projection techniques should be used only for short-range forecasts, the next one or two time periods at most.

Chapter 4 describes the simplest of projection techniques, linear extrapolation. All extrapolation projections extend past patterns unchanged into the future. Three forms of extrapolation are discussed. The first employs visual examination of plots of past utilization. The second uses simple mathematics to calculate mean amounts of change between periods. The third is the familiar and commonly used statistical tool, the simple linear regression. Complex forms of this basic tool are identified, though few are examined in detail because they would require computer rather than do-it-yourself application.

Chapter 5 covers a slightly more complex projection technique called *autocorrelation*. Where linear extrapolation extends the complete past pattern into the future, autocorrelation bases its projection on the most recent period. The relationship between each period and its preceding period is the pattern projected rather than a pattern that describes all the past periods at once. Three forms of autocorrelation are examined. A graphic technique identifies a mean slope between periods. The mathematical technique calculates a mean rate of change between periods. An autoregression is the counterpart to the simple linear regression.

Chapter 6 covers analytic techniques that modify past patterns rather than extrapolate them unchanged. An exponential smoothing approach incorporates a way of giving greater weight to more recent than more distant utilization experience. Moving averages techniques separate extreme fluctuations from basic underlying trends in past utilization data. Time series analysis breaks down past utilization observations into cycles, trends, and unexplained variation and uses both past cycles and past trends to project future utilization.

Chapter 7 identifies two projection techniques based on marketing concepts. An innovation adoption or diffusion curve fits past utilization data to a complex S-shaped curve or ogive that has been found to characterize patterns of growth in innovative behavior. It projects based on directly relevant past data and the history of similar cases or analogs. Intention surveys rely on asking people how they intend to behave with respect to health services utilization. It relies on both expressed intention and past histories of the reliability of such experience.

# Chapter 4

# Linear Extrapolation

A linear extrapolation approach to forecasting entails describing the pattern of past utilization as a linear function. The line may be drawn graphically, using visual judgment as to its form and proximity to plotted observations. The line may also be described in terms of an arithmetic function, an average rate or amount of change characterizing past observations. Finally, the line may be calculated as a statistical function called a *linear regression,* in which the dependent variable is a quantity of utilization and the independent or predictive variable is a unit of time.

## GRAPHIC EXTRAPOLATION

The use of drawn lines to project utilization is a relatively simple example of the extrapolation technique. It requires only the plotting of past utilization data on a volume–time matrix and a draftsman's skills in drawing a line that comes as close as possible to the plotted data points. It is typically used to provide basic insights into the likely mathematical form of a projection pattern, though it can be employed on its own as a forecasting device.

Plotting of utilization data may be done on standard or logarithmic graphic paper. Examples of how a plot might look are given in Figures 4-1 through 4-4.

Figure 4-1 suggests a fairly strong linear pattern or trend in observed utilization. A straight line could easily be drawn so as to keep roughly an equal number of plotted observations above and below it. Such a line would have a definite upward slope and project increasing utilization over time. The "fit" of the line would be judged by how far on the average each plotted point is from the line.

**Figure 4-1** Linear Pattern

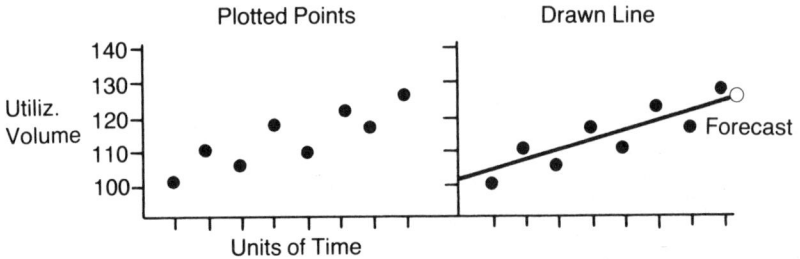

Because the line as a whole is used to project future utilization, the forecast for next period's volume is actually less than the observed volume this period despite the upward trend. This is due to the variability of actual observations about the apparent trend. The most recent period is substantially above the trend, more than the slope of the line projects as an increase from one period to the next.

Figure 4-2 displays a curvilinear trend rather than a straight line. Again in keeping an equal number of observations above and below the curve, an estimate of the curvilinear trend could easily be drawn as shown. A compass or draftsman's french curve may be used as a guide to drawing the best curve. The curve shown illustrates one of the risks inherent in curvilinear extrapolations. It projects dramatically increasing utilization in the next five periods and tends to forecast infinity quickly. Such a curve is actually observed at the beginning of an innovation adoption pattern (see Chapter 7).

Figure 4-3 illustrates a plot pattern in which no clear trend is visible. A pattern with absolutely no measurable trend is actually quite rare if analyzed statistically. The illustrated pattern would produce a poor fit with any trend drawn, however. In such a case, estimating the future as the *mean* of past observations is the safest practice. If the reasons for such a strange pattern are known, however, and confident estimates of future changes can be developed, some forecast other than the mean may be appropriate.

Figure 4-4 portrays a cyclical pattern. Such patterns are fairly common in health services utilization where seasonal patterns of population (resort areas) or disease (upper respiratory infections in winter, greater trauma in summer) are present. A plot of weekly census in a hospital would show a recurring cycle of high levels in the middle of the week followed by low levels on weekends and holidays. High utilization of emergency rooms may reflect weekly paydays, weekends, full moon, or a variety of recurrent factors. Where regular repeating peaks and troughs occur at consistent intervals, a cyclical extrapolation works best. (Cycles are discussed further in Chapter 6 and Chapter 14.)

It is a good practice, when considering a linear extrapolation technique for forecasting, to plot past data on graph paper first. A plot on conventional paper is a good first step with semilog and full log paper a subsequent possibility. A semilog plot, for example, would smooth out the curve in

**Figure 4-2** Curvilinear Pattern

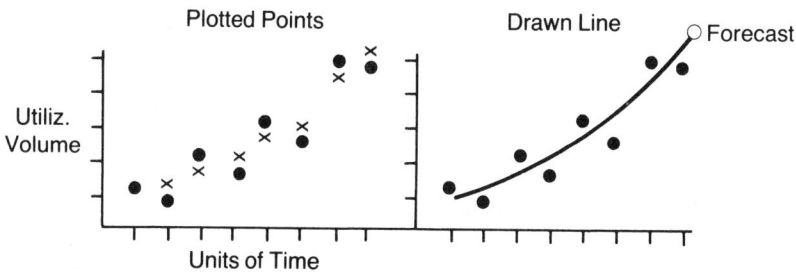

**Figure 4-3** No Pattern

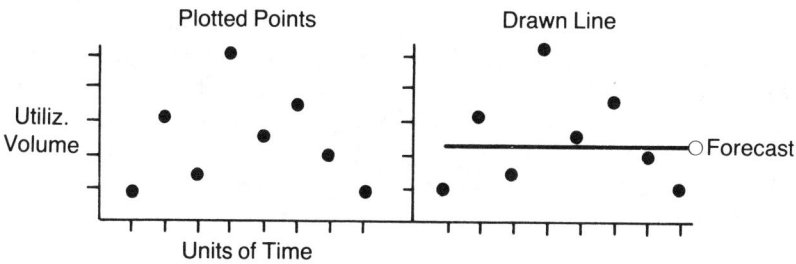

**Figure 4-4** Cyclical Pattern

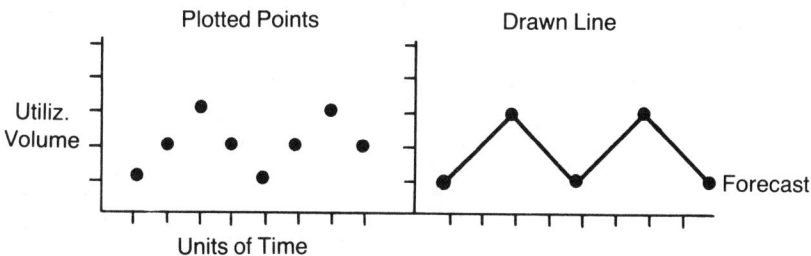

Figure 4-2 and make it easier to draw a straight line as an extrapolator. The plot of past data contributes two useful bits of information to the forecaster. It indicates the form of the pattern present in past data, and it suggests how many periods of data are required to measure that pattern mathematically. A cyclical pattern, for example, typically requires much more data to measure than a linear one, with a curvilinear pattern somewhere between the two.


**AVERAGE CHANGE**

    The simplest mathematical approaches to linear extrapolation involve calculating average change levels in past utilization data. The choice lies between employing an arithmetic or geometric approach. An arithmetic choice calculates the average *amount* of change present in observed utilization. The geometric choice calculates the average rate of change. If a plot of past data suggests a straight-line trend, the average amount approach is preferred. If past utilization forms a curve, the average rate would be a better device.

    The data in Table 4-1 might reflect past numbers of monthly visits to a clinic, for example. A true linear extrapolation based on these data begins with the mean value for the entire past sequence, or 4,698 in this case. The mean is used so that no single period exerts more influence than any other on the extrapolation. The mean corresponds to what should be the utilization for the midpoint in the sequence, or period $(1 + 8) \div 2 = 4.5$. Thus the projection for period 9 would be equal to the mean plus $(9 - 4.5) = 4.5$ periods times the average amount of change, or $4,697.8 + 4.5 (84.3) = 5,077.2$. Using the most recent period as a starting point would produce a far different result, i.e., $4,925 + 84.3 = 5,009.3$. Beginning with the

**Table 4-1** Monthly Clinic Visits

| Period | Visits | Change |
|--------|--------|--------|
| 1 | 4,335 | +153 |
| 2 | 4,488 | + 74 |
| 3 | 4,562 | +167 |
| 4 | 4,729 | + 73 |
| 5 | 4,802 | + 49 |
| 6 | 4,851 | + 39 |
| 7 | 4,890 | + 35 |
| 8 | 4,925 | |
| Mean | 4,697.8 | + 84.3 |

latest period, however, is an autocorrelation form of projection rather than a linear extrapolation (see Chapter 5).

The data in this example suggest that the amount of change from one period to the next is diminishing with each period. If so, an average *rate* of change approach would be preferred. With the same data, rates of change between periods are shown in Table 4-2.

A curvilinear extrapolation would begin with the mean and multiply it by 1.018 for midpoint-minus-one periods. A projection for period 9 would be 4,698 as if invested at 1.8 percent interest compounded over $9 - 4.5 = 4.5$ periods. That would equal $4,698 \times 1.018^{4.5} = 4,698 \times 1.08359 = 5,090.7$.

An average amount- or rate-of-change approach can be an adequate projection technique if the pattern of changes in observed data is a fairly simple one and if it is used, as all projection techniques should be, for short-term forecasts. Where more complex patterns are present, i.e., where the amounts or rates of change are changing in some patterned way, more complex projection techniques should be used. Because changes in rates or amounts of change per period suggest changing dynamics, it would be a good idea to investigate why such changes have occurred rather than blindly projecting future utilization.

## LINEAR REGRESSION

A simple linear regression is the statistical counterpart to the average amount of change approach. With inexpensive handheld calculators capable of performing such regressions, it is virtually as easy to employ this technique as to use the arithmetic alternative. With the same data as in

**Table 4-2**  Rates of Change

| Period | Visits | Change (2 ÷ 1, etc.) |
|---|---|---|
| 1 | 4,335 | |
| 2 | 4,488 | 1.035 |
| 3 | 4,562 | 1.016 |
| 4 | 4,729 | 1.037 |
| 5 | 4,802 | 1.015 |
| 6 | 4,851 | 1.010 |
| 7 | 4,890 | 1.008 |
| 8 | 4,925 | 1.007 |
| Mean | 4,697.8 | 1.018 |

the previous illustrations, for example, a linear regression would produce the following result:

$$
\begin{aligned}
\text{correlation } (r) &= .9687 \\
\text{coefficient of determination } (r^2) &= .9384 \\
\text{intercept } (a) &= 4{,}318.5 \\
\text{slope } (b) &= 84.3
\end{aligned}
$$

Because calculators vary greatly from one to another, no standard instructions on performing a linear regression on a calculator can be offered. The typical approach for a time series extrapolation requires merely punching in a 1 as the independent variable once, followed by the data for period 1 as the independent. Data for subsequent periods are then added in order until all periods' data have been punched in. After that, correlation, slope, and intercept buttons are pushed, with the correlation value then squared to yield the coefficient of determination.

The form of a linear regression used for a time series extrapolation is

$$
\begin{aligned}
u &= a + b(t) \\
\text{where } u &= \text{utilization} \\
a &= \text{intercept} \\
b &= \text{coefficient or slope} \\
t &= \text{the number of the time period}
\end{aligned}
$$

The goodness of fit of past data is reflected in the coefficient of determination, or $r^2$. With a value of .9384, the illustrated regression suggests a good fit indeed. The statistical significance of the regression is indicated by the $F$ statistic. This test statistic is a function of the value of $r^2$ and the number of observations in the regression. In a time series regression, the $F$ statistic is calculated as follows:

$$
F = \frac{r^2(n - 1)}{1 - r^2}
$$

or in this case

$$
F = \frac{(.9384)(7)}{.0616} = 106.6
$$

The $F$ statistic is then looked up in an $F$ statistic table in some statistical text under 1, $n - 1$ degrees of freedom. In this case the $F$ statistic meets the most stringent standard because it suggests that the chances are less than 1 percent ($p < .01$) that such a high $r^2$ value could have occurred by chance alone. The $r^2$ and $F$ test values describe only how well the regression *described the past*, of course, and *do not* indicate their potential for forecasting the future. Only a confident belief in the persistence of the observed pattern suggests the value of a regression in forecasting.

The forecast of period 9 resulting from this regression would be 4,318.5 + 84.3(9) = 5,077.2. (This is the same as the average amount of change projection.) It calculates an imaginary value for period 0 or the period before the utilization data examined, then adds a standard amount for each subsequent period. It is an average amount of change approach. In this case it produces a forecast in keeping with those resulting from the simpler arithmetic techniques but not in keeping with the observation that the amount of change had been diminishing over time.

Because both the amounts and rates of change in the example are clearly diminishing, it would seem a good idea to try regressing the changes rather than the utilization volume itself. A regression of the amounts of change, i.e., +153, +74, +167, +73, +49, +39, +35, would produce the following results:

$$r = .774$$
$$r^2 = .599$$
$$a = 161.7$$
$$b = -19.4$$

Because the mean utilization level occurs in the (1 + 8) ÷ 2 = 4.5th period, the projection for the 9th period would be the mean, 4,697.8, plus the regression predicted 4.5th, 5th, 6th, 7th, and 8th changes, or 4,697.8 + 74.6 + 64.9 + 45.6 + 26.2 + 6.9 = 4,916. (One of the delights of a modern calculator is that it can do things like calculate the expected change for the 4.5th period, when paper and pencil would have a difficult time.) This projection at least reflects the pattern of diminishing changes in utilization where a regression of the volume data themselves does not.

A rate of change regression for the change data would produce the following:

$$r = .780$$
$$r^2 = .608$$
$$a = 1.036$$
$$b = -.0045$$

Predicted 4.5th, 5th, 6th, 7th, and 8th changes are 1.016, 1.014, 1.009,

1.005, 1.00014, so the projection for period 9 would be 4,697.8 × 1.016 × 1.014 × 1.009 × 1.005 × 1.00014 = 4,908.5. By regressing the rates of change, the projection more accurately reflects the pattern of diminishing changes.

The $r^2$ values for the regressions of change (.774 and .780) are less than the $r^2$ value for the regression of the utilization data themselves (.938). In spite of this the change regressions clearly do a better job of describing the pattern of utilization changes than the utilization regression does. A linear regression has to use a uniform amount of change from period to period. By separating out the actual changes, a better pattern is identified. In general, identifying and examining the pattern of changes in utilization over time, i.e., the differences between utilization levels from one period to another, mean a better basis for linear extrapolation.

In regard to the $r^2$ value, mathematically the $r^2$ value describes how much closer a linear (or log-linear) regression comes to matching observations than would estimating each observation as the mean of all. It tends to be high when observations deviate greatly from the mean, i.e., where there is a significant slope to the data, even though data might deviate greatly from the trend line also. Thus the $r^2$ value is likely to be high in cases such as the example used in this chapter, even though the linear regression does not do a particularly good job of describing change patterns. Because the data did follow a significant trend, the regression did far better at matching the data than would the mean as an estimator for each period's utilization. As a projection tool, however, the regression of the utilization data is far inferior to the regression of the changes in terms of accurately reflecting those changes.

Another caution about $r^2$ values. This value describes the success of the regression in matching past data but has nothing to do with its likelihood of accurately anticipating the future. In Chapter 3 the $r^2$ values of over 150 regressions were tested against their forecasting accuracy. The results indicated that, if anything, the $r^2$ value was *negatively* correlated with forecasting accuracy. This reflects the fact that steep slopes in past data tend to produce high $r^2$ values but tend not to persevere in the real world. This same test indicated that the last year of a time series was a better forecaster of subsequent utilization than the regression of previous years was.

The linear regression equivalent of the average rate of change approach is the log-linear regression. The logarithms for each utilization calculation are first calculated, then these log-values are regressed in a time series. With calculators easily capable of supplying log-values for each observation, this approach is only slightly more complicated than the simple linear regression. The data in Table 4-3 illustrate this. This is virtually the same as the rate of change projection.

Even this log-linear regression fails to take into account the declining rate of increase that characterizes the data. If an average amount of change analysis were made of the logarithms for observed utilization, a projection of log $= 3.637 + (8)(.008) = 3.701$ would result for period 9. The antilog of this projection, i.e., $10^{3.701} = 5,023$, is in contrast to the regression prediction of 5,092. An average rate of change approach applied to the logarithms would produce a log of $3.637 \times 1.0021^8 = 3.699$ for period 9, hence a forecast of $10^{3.699} = 4,995$ for the period.

In recognizing that there is a pattern in the fact that both rates and amounts of changes are diminishing, a regression could be performed of the changes. A regression of the seven *amounts* of change, for example, would predict that the eighth change will be a minus change or decrease of .00196. Applying this to the logarithms would mean that the log for period 9 should be $3.692 - .00196 = 3.690$ and the forecast, $10^{3.690} = 4,898$. A regression of the *rates* of change would suggest that the rate for the eighth change would be $.99998571 \times 3.692 = 3.6919$, and the forecast would be $10^{3.6919} = 4,920$ visits.

These whimsical manipulations are designed to illustrate the range of possibilities inherent in linear extrapolation. Only judgment can decide which ought to be used in forecasting or whether linear extrapolation is a

---

**Table 4-3** Log-Linear Regression

| Period | Utilization Data | Log | Change Rate | Change Amount |
|--------|-----------------|------|------|--------|
| 1 | 4,335 | 3.637 | | |
| 2 | 4,488 | 3.652 | 1.0041 | +.015 |
| 3 | 4,562 | 3.659 | 1.0019 | +.007 |
| 4 | 4,729 | 3.675 | 1.0044 | +.016 |
| 5 | 4,802 | 3.681 | 1.0016 | +.006 |
| 6 | 4,857 | 3.686 | 1.0014 | +.005 |
| 7 | 4,890 | 3.689 | 1.0008 | +.003 |
| 8 | 4,925 | 3.692 | 1.0008 | +.003 |
| | | | Mean 1.0021 | +.008 |

$r$ = .9653
$r^2$ = .9317
intercept = 3.636
slope = .00787
forecast for period 9 = antilog 3.707 or 5,092

sensible choice at all. The technique that best fits past data is probably the best choice where there is a rational confidence that the dynamics responsible for the pattern of past utilization will behave in the same fashion through the period to be forecast. In the preceding illustration, the best forecast based on common-sense examination of the data would be based on an expectation that the amount of change between the eighth and ninth periods will be around 20 to 25, and the ninth period should be about 4,945 to 4,950. The same type of examination applied to the rates of change in the past data would produce an expectation that the next rate of change should be around 1.005, and the ninth period, 1.005 × 4,925, or 4,949.6, close to the amount of change prediction.

Visual examination of the observed utilization levels, and of the plotted data points, should be a routine part of any forecasting effort. Mathematical and statistical techniques can impose patterns as part of the technique, even if such patterns don't really describe the behavior of past data. Good, common-sense judgment should always be employed together with or even instead of mere calculation.

## SUMMARY

Linear extrapolation begins by identifying the pattern that best describes what has been happening in past utilization, then projects that pattern into the future. Graphic techniques accomplish this visually by plotting observations on a graph and drawing a line as close as possible to the plotted points. It is used primarily to provide a visual clue to the mathematical or statistical tool that will do the best job in describing the pattern.

Mathematical extrapolation identifies the amount or rates of change from period to period in past utilization. The average amount or rate of change is then identified and used to project future period values. By identifying the amounts and rates of change between periods, more complex patterns of utilization may be developed, suggesting more complex projection techniques. If the amounts or rates of change are observed to be uniform, they may be used to make projections without further analysis.

A linear regression essentially replicates the mathematical approaches but also provides specific measures of how well observations fit the identified pattern. Generally speaking, the better the fit, the better the pattern identified, though only in terms of describing the past. The fit of the regression to past data is only correlated with good forecasting accuracy when the dynamics producing past changes persevere unchanged. In general, regressions of the *changes* between periods do a better job of matching past data than a regression of the utilization data themselves does.

When considering the use of an extrapolation technique, it is a good idea to keep in mind one of Mark Twain's stories. Although it applies specifically to the extrapolation of past trends, it includes a warning relative to the scientific versus conjectural nature of forecasting in general:

> In the space of one hundred and seventy-six years the Lower Mississippi has shortened itself two hundred and forty-two miles. That is an average of a trifle over one mile and a third per year. Therefore, any calm person, who is not blind or idiotic, can see that in the old Oolitic Silurian Period, just a million years ago next November, the Lower Mississippi River was upward of one million three hundred thousand miles long, and stuck out over the Gulf of Mexico like a fishing rod. And by the same token any person can see that seven hundred and forty-two years from now the Lower Mississippi will be only a mile and three-quarters long, and Cairo and New Orleans will have joined their streets together, and be plodding comfortably along under a single mayor and a mutual board of aldermen. There is something fascinating about science. One gets such wholesome returns of conjecture out of such trifling investment of fact. *(Life on the Mississippi).*

---

**Annotated Bibliography**

**Donlon, V.** "Statistical Methods to Forecast Volume of Service for the Revenue Budget." *Hospital Financial Management* 5, no. 4 (April 1975): 38.
    Discusses use of linear regression to forecast utilization and revenues in a hospital.

**Feldstein, P., and German, J.** "Predicting Hospital Utilization: An Evaluation of Three Approaches." *Inquiry* 2, no. 1 (Winter 1965): 13.
    Evaluates simple linear regression compared to causal alternatives in predicting statewide hospital use rates.

**Fildes, R.** "Quantitative Forecasting—The State of the Art: Extrapolative Models." *Journal of the Operations Research Society* 30, no. 8 (1979): 691.
    Discusses range of extrapolation techniques available for forecasting, from simple trending through smoothing and time series models, reaching no conclusions as to which technique is generally superior.

**Griffith, J.** *Quantitative Techniques for Hospital Planning and Control.* Lexington, MA: Lexington Books, 1972.
    Part I contains an excellent introduction to the linear regression in forecasting demand.

**Tummins, M., et al.** "Regression Analysis—How to Apply It in Managing Costs." *Hospital Financial Management* 8, no. 12 (December 1978): 28.
    Discusses the use of simple linear regression in forecasting utilization for budgeting and cost control.

**Walker, L., and Greenwald, E.** "Two Simple Accurate Forecasting Models." *Hospital Financial Management* 8, no. 3 (March 1978): 16.
    Discusses average amount and rate of change approaches.

# Chapter 5

# Autocorrelation

Where linear extrapolation techniques rely on lines linking all past data together, autocorrelation employs the relationship between utilization data from one period and the data from a single prior period. A large number of such pairs should be examined to identify the nature and strength of this correlation. Once identified, the correlation measure or ratio is used to project utilization on the basis of some recently observed utilization. Like linear extrapolation, autocorrelation projections can be derived through graphics, averaging changes, or statistical regression.

Two choices apply in all autocorrelation analyses, related to the selection of pairs of utilization data. The first is the choice between using pairs of data from immediately adjacent periods or selecting pairs from time-lagged periods. The second is the choice between using data from periods of the same length or data from unequal periods.

*Adjacent versus time-lagged* choices may be made for analytic or convenience reasons. If there is a clear cycle present in the data, utilization in a given period might be more closely and consistently related to utilization 2, 3, or even 5 or 10 periods before the immediately preceding period. This does not mean that utilization from time-lagged periods should be identical or similar, merely that they be related in a consistent fashion. If utilization in one period is consistently 10 percent greater than that of utilization 5 periods before, then the correlation between them is 1.10 to 1.00, and the consistency of that ratio is what makes it a good projection device.

Besides choosing adjacent or time-lagged periods for reasons of consistency, there may be a convenience reason to choose time lagging. If the forecasting task is to estimate utilization for next month and the forecast must be developed in the middle of this month, then it might be best to look for the ratio between utilization levels separated by one month. That way it will be possible to use the known utilization from last month to forecast next month. Otherwise the forecast would have to be based on an estimate of this month's utilization rather than true experience.

Similar versus dissimilar period choices are likely to be made for the same reasons, though convenience is likely to dominate. In the preceding example, if it is necessary to forecast next month's utilization after experiencing only 10 days of this month, then the autocorrelation ratio chosen for analysis could be that between the first 10 days of each month and the full month following. Adjustments would have to be made for months of different length and for cases where some 10-day periods include two weekends versus one, or holidays, for example.

There is an important requirement in autocorrelation projection relative to the data used to identify past relationships. The relationship that is used to project utilization should be the same relationship that is analyzed in the past. If estimates of this year's utilization available in July are to be used in forecasting next year's utilization, then the *estimates* made in previous Julys relative to their following years should be what is analyzed in the past. The correlation between actual year's utilization and the following year may be stronger, i.e., more consistent, but might not be the best description of the relationship between July's estimate and the following year.

Generally speaking, it is best to avoid using estimates at all as the basis for forecasting. If a forecast of next year's utilization must be made after only six months' experience with this year, the best autocorrelation to analyze would be that between utilization in the first six months of past years and that of the following full years. Because unequal periods can be used in autocorrelation and where there is a consistent and hopefully persistent relationship between dissimilar periods, this approach tends to work better than using estimates. (See Chapter 16 for a specific application of dissimilar period correlations.)

## GRAPHIC AUTOCORRELATION

Because autocorrelation links utilization in one period to utilization in a single prior period, the purpose of graphic analysis is to portray the sorts of relationships that have existed among past pairs of periods. Because only two points are involved in each pair, the relationship can be portrayed only as a straight line. Although other types of lines could be drawn, only the straight line is an unbiased description of the relationship.

Autocorrelation graphics draw lines between each member of the selected pairs as plotted. In Figure 5-1, for example, the dots are connected, showing a fairly typical pattern.

The fact that the lines run at widely dissimilar angles suggests that there is little consistency in the relationship between data in adjacent periods. In such a case time lagging might be employed to see if staggering the periods produces a more consistent relationship. Figure 5-2 shows a time-lagged graphic analysis of the same data with a one-period separation. This analysis produces a different picture entirely. It suggests that the relationship between the time-lagged pairs is quite consistent, where adjacent pairs are inconsistent. Such a result would strongly suggest the use of time lagging for analytical reasons, whether or not convenience is a consideration.

As with linear extrapolation, a graphic approach to autocorrelation can be used to project utilization by itself. In the preceding example the projection for the next time period, period 11, would start with the data

**Figure 5-1** Autocorrelation Graphics

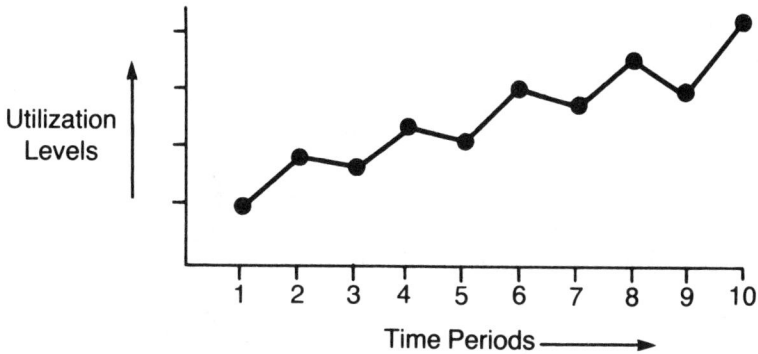

**Figure 5-2** Time-Lagged Analysis

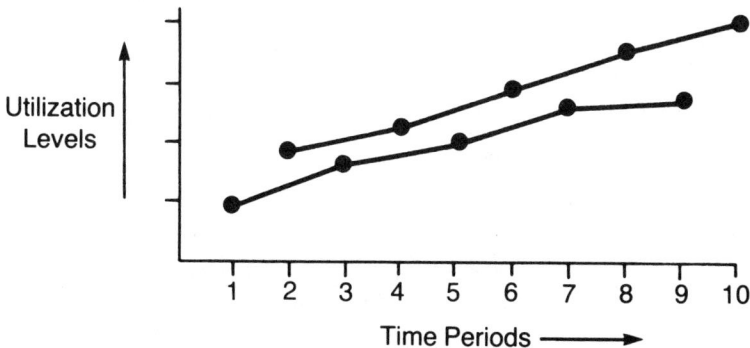

from period 9 and project a modest increase. To estimate the average relationship graphically between past time-lagged periods, the lines connecting past periods may be superimposed, as in Figure 5-3. The average angle may then be visually estimated and applied to the ninth period.

More often, however, the graphic examination of autocorrelation is used to determine whether the technique shows promise. It also serves to suggest whether time lagging might be better than use of adjacent periods. It can also be used to judge whether the relationship between dissimilar periods is promising as a forecasting tool, as shown in Figure 5-4. If any alternative appears promising, a mathematical or statistical approach would then be used actually to develop the projection.

**Figure 5-3** Average Relationship between Past Time-Lagged Periods

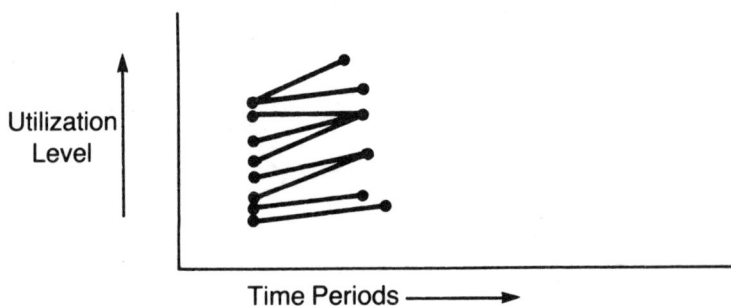

**Figure 5-4** Relationship between Dissimilar Periods

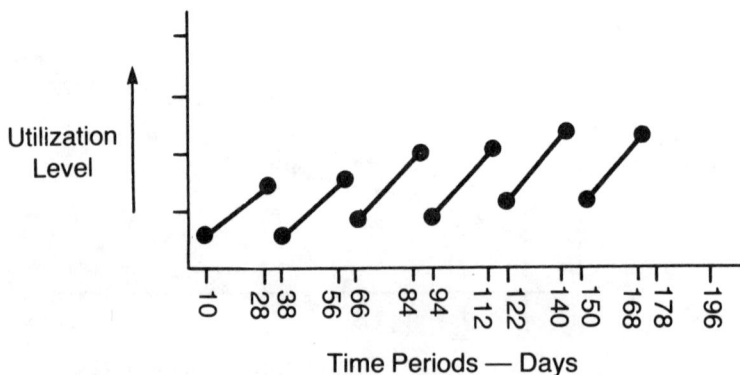

Figure 5-4 shows the relationships between the first 10 days of 28-day periods and the entire 28-day period. Such an approach can be used to forecast utilization for full four-week periods after only the first 10 days' experience. The use of 28-day accounting periods eliminates the vagaries of monthly time frames, though some adjustments might have to be made for holidays.

## MATHEMATICAL AUTOCORRELATION

Like linear extrapolation, mathematical approaches to autocorrelation can employ either amount or rate of change between periods to describe past relationships. The amounts or rates can be applied to adjacent or time-lagged periods of equal or unequal length. It is the consistency of such amounts or rates that affects the use of autocorrelation in projecting utilization.

The data in Table 5-1 illustrate the application of autocorrelation analysis. Once the average amount or rate of change prevalent in past data has been identified, it is then applied to the most recent period. This is where it differs from the linear extrapolation approach, which applies average changes to the mean of the entire past time period rather than the most recent period. Linear extrapolation relies on a pattern covering all past data periods where autocorrelation looks at individual pairs, hence takes off from the most recent experience.

In the preceding example both graphic analysis and visual examination of the amounts and rates of change would suggest the appropriateness of

**Table 5-1** Application of Autocorrelation Analysis

| Period | Utilization | Change Amount | Rate |
|--------|-------------|---------------|------|
| 1 | 600 | | |
| | | +200 | 1.333 |
| 2 | 800 | | |
| | | − 2 | .998 |
| 3 | 798 | | |
| | | +266 | 1.333 |
| 4 | 1,064 | | |
| | | − 3 | .997 |
| 5 | 1,061 | | |
| | | +354 | 1.334 |
| 6 | 1,415 | | |
| | | − 3 | .998 |
| 7 | 1,412 | | |
| | | +470 | 1.333 |
| 8 | 1,882 | | |
| | | − 4 | .998 |
| 9 | 1,878 | | |
| Mean | | 159.8 | 1.165 |

time lagging. The amounts and rates of change between time-lagged pairs separated by one period would be as shown in Table 5-2.

The rate of change is clearly the more consistent of the two. In order to predict utilization for period 10, the time-lagged autocorrelation would begin with utilization in period 8, then multiply it by 1.330, the mean rate of change. The result would be 1,882 × 1.330 = 2,503. The forecast for period 11 would be period 9 utilization times the same rates of change, i.e., 1,878 × 1.330 = 2,497.

The careful forecaster would certainly wish to understand why such a pattern prevailed in past data before relying on it to project utilization. The data might represent utilization of the mining company's employee clinic per week, for example. The rate of growth is accounted for by the fact that the number of employees is increasing by one-third every two weeks. The strange pattern of high use increase followed by stability could be due to a requirement that all new workers come in for a physical their first week on the job. It might also be due to paying workers every two weeks, followed by their requiring health care to recover from the effects of celebrating. The choice of whether to rely on the past pattern should be governed by good information on the intentions of the company. Will it be adding a third more employees and will it continue to pay workers every two weeks or require first-week physicals? If any of the factors explaining the past pattern change, the projection relying on that pattern is likely to be erroneous.

## AUTOREGRESSION

The statistical counterpart of the linear regression in autocorrelation is autoregression. It is simply the statistically determined and assessed relationship between utilization in one period and that of another, whether

**Table 5-2** Time-Lagged Pairs Separated by One Period

| Period Pair | Amount | Rate |
|:---:|:---:|---:|
| 1–3 | 198 | 1.330 |
| 2–4 | 264 | 1.330 |
| 3–5 | 263 | 1.330 |
| 4–6 | 351 | 1.330 |
| 5–7 | 351 | 1.331 |
| 6–8 | 467 | 1.330 |
| 7–9 | 466 | 1.330 |
| Mean | 337.1 | 1.330 |

adjacent or time-lagged, equal or unequal in length. The advantage of autoregression lies chiefly in its greater apparent sophistication and its ability to offer statistical measures of past fit between the data and the identified pattern.

An autoregression can be easily calculated on a preprogrammed calculator. The preceding period data, i.e., the independent variable, is entered first, then the subsequent period data or dependent variable is entered. At least 5 and preferably 10 pairs of data inputs should be employed to assess the correlation and its consistency. The correlation itself is expressed as a mathematical function representing the best way to project a subsequent period's utilization given that of a preceding period. The calculator also calculates the correlation coefficient reflecting the consistency of the relationship ($r$), from which the coefficient of determination may be calculated ($r^2$), and the standard deviation of the dependent variable observations, from which the standard deviation of the regression can be calculated.

An autoregression based on the adjacent period series—600, 800, 798, 1,064, 1,061, 1,415, 1,412, 1,882, 1,878—would produce the following result:

$$
\begin{aligned}
r &= .901 \\
r^2 &= .812 \\
a &= 240.1 \\
b &= .9288
\end{aligned}
$$

The formula for an autoregression is

$$\text{utilization}_{(t + 1)} = a + b \times \text{utilization}_{(t)}$$

Thus the prediction for the 10th period would be 240.1 + .9288(1,878), or 1,984.4.

For comparison, a linear regression of the same data would produce the following results:

$$
\begin{aligned}
r &= .974 \\
r^2 &= .949 \\
a &= 384.1 \\
b &= 165.6
\end{aligned}
$$

The formula for the linear regression would be

$$\text{utilization}_{(t)} = a + b_{(t)}$$

so its forecast of utilization for period 10 would be

$$384.1 + 10(165.6) = 2,040.1$$

Applying time lagging to the same data would analyze the pairs in Table 5-3. The results of the time-lagged autocorrelation would be as follows:

$$
\begin{aligned}
r &= .9999996 \\
r^2 &= .9999992 \\
a &= -0.173 \\
b &= 1.330
\end{aligned}
$$

The formula for this time-lagged correlation would be

$$U_{(t+2)} = a + b_{(U_t)}$$

To predict utilization for period 10, the data for period 8 rather than period 9 would be used, and the projected utilization would be

$$-0.173 + 1.330(1,878) = 2,498$$

The extremely high $r^2$ value in this regression indicates an extraordinary fit with the past data. The limits of the $r^2$ value in assessing the forecasting ability of a regression are clearly shown by the fact that the simple adjacent period linear regression had a $r^2$ value of .949, ordinarily a delightfully high value. Yet its projection for the next period's utilization is 2,040.3 versus the time-lagged autoregression projection of 2,498, 22.4 percent higher. The adjacent period autocorrelation had a high $r^2$ value, i.e., .812

**Table 5-3** Utilization Periods

| Periods | Utilization |
|---------|-------------|
| 1–3 | 600– 798 |
| 2–4 | 800–1,064 |
| 3–5 | 798–1,061 |
| 4–6 | 1,064–1,415 |
| 5–7 | 1,061–1,412 |
| 6–8 | 1,415–1,882 |
| 7–9 | 1,412–1,878 |

and projected the next period's utilization as 1,984.4. There is likely to be little relationship between $r^2$ values themselves and forecasting accuracy in practice. The $r^2$ value simply shows which pattern does the best job of describing past utilization without indicating how well in absolute terms the pattern will predict the future.

The formula for an autoregression indicates the type of relationship that exists across the pairs of utilization data examined. Where the relationship is linear, i.e., where the amount of change between adjacent or time-lagged periods is relatively stable, the *intercept* is large relative to the utilization data, and the slope is close to 1.000. A perfectly linear or arithmetical relationship, where the *amount* of difference between observed pairs is always the same, would produce a regression with the intercept equal to the difference and the slope equal to 1.000.

In contrast, where the relationship between observations is close to a constant rate of change, the intercept is relatively small and the slope different from 1.000. In a case where the rate of change across adjacent or time-lagged periods is always the same, the slope is that rate of change and the intercept is zero. Where either the slope is close to 1.000 or the intercept close to zero, the $r$ and $r^2$ values tend to be high. When neither situation holds, the $r$ and $r^2$ values are lower.

## UNEQUAL PERIODS

It is not at all necessary for autocorrelations to be between utilization levels in periods of equal length. Some inequality is unavoidable if month-to-month correlations are used, for example, and there is even a slight inequality in year-to-year relationship because of leap year. As long as a *consistent* relationship can be found, fairly precise estimates of the future can be developed based on correlations between unequal periods.

Examination of past utilization might well reveal that utilization levels on Friday of one week are consistently related to the utilization during the entire week that follows. Utilization during November might prove consistently related to utilization during the entire year that follows. The only way it can be ascertained if such consistent relationships exist is to examine potential relationships to see whether they are consistent.

The data in Table 5-4 might represent utilization volumes for November versus the entire following year, for example.

If November of this year has 2,014 utilization volume, then the utilization for next year ought to be close to 2,014 ÷ .08688 = 23,181, based on the preceding relationship. The consistency of that relationship can be seen

**Table 5-4** Utilization Volumes

| Period | (1)<br>November | (2)<br>Next Year | Ratio (1 ÷ 2) |
|---|---|---|---|
| 1 | 1,436 | 16,514 | .08696 |
| 2 | 1,382 | 15,755 | .08772 |
| 3 | 1,578 | 18,305 | .08621 |
| 4 | 1,632 | 18,605 | .08772 |
| 5 | 1,513 | 17,399 | .08696 |
| 6 | 1,491 | 17,296 | .08620 |
| 7 | 1,550 | 18,167 | .08532 |
| 8 | 1,604 | 18,125 | .08850 |
| 9 | 1,692 | 19,289 | .08772 |
| 10 | 1,747 | 20,440 | .08547 |
| | | Mean | .08688 |

by simply examining how close all the ratios are to the mean value. It can also be calculated via autoregression, with the following results:

$$
\begin{aligned}
r &= .986 \\
r^2 &= .972 \\
\text{intercept} &= -395.8 \\
\text{slope} &= 11.7666 \\
\text{mean} &= 17,989.5 \\
\text{standard deviation} &= 1,342.5
\end{aligned}
$$

The formula for the regression would be

$$\text{utilization}_{(\text{whole year})} = -395.8 + 11.7666(\text{utilization}_{(\text{November})})$$

so

$$-395.8 + 11.7666(2,014) = 23,302$$

would be the regression-projected forecast for next year based on this November.

The precision of the forecast would be estimated as follows:

$$
\begin{aligned}
\text{standard deviation}_{(\text{regression})} &= \sqrt{(\text{standard deviation}_{(\text{observation})})^2 \times 1 - r^2} \\
&= \sqrt{(1,342.5)^2 \times 1 - .972} \\
&= \sqrt{1,802,306.3 \times .028} \\
&= 224.6
\end{aligned}
$$

precision                           = $\dfrac{\text{standard deviation of regression}}{\text{mean of observations}}$

$= \dfrac{224.6}{17,989.5} = .0125$

confidence interval          = $\pm\ 1.96(.0125) = \pm\ 2.45\%$

Such precision is likely to be excellent for most purposes, especially when compared to the estimated precision available through other projection and forecasting techniques. It still depends on the perseverance of past patterns, as do all projection forecasts.

## PRECISION ESTIMATES

A key to assessing the value of a regression, whether a linear regression or an autoregression, is its precision. The precision of a regression is indicated by its standard deviation. The ratio between the standard deviation of the regression and the mean of past observation yields a good precision measure. The confidence interval of a regression forecast is usually plus or minus 1.96 standard deviations from the forecast. If the regression accurately portrays the future as well as the past, i.e., if the relationship on which it rests persists unchanged, future observations should be within plus or minus 1.96 standard deviations 19 times of 20, or 95 percent of the time.

If decisions are more sensitive to future utilization being *less* than predicted, the forecaster may worry only about potential deviation below the projection. A 95 percent confidence level for the projection can be set at 1.645 standard deviations below the mean. In the previous example, the mean of the observations was 1,358.6 (this is the mean of all dependent variables, the second entry in each correlation pair). The standard deviation of the *observations* is 416.2. This is not the standard deviation of interest, however, because it simply describes the pattern of deviation of all dependent variables from their mean.

To calculate the standard deviation of the *regression,* indicating how close it comes to describing past relationships, two approaches may be used. The regression can be used to *predict* the value of each dependent variable, given the independent. Then the predicted values can be compared to actual observations, and the standard deviation computed in the traditional manner as the square root of the sum of all squared deviations divided by one less than the number of observed pairs, i.e.,

$$\text{standard deviation} = \sqrt{\frac{\Sigma(\text{obs.} - \text{pred.})^2}{n - 1}}$$

For the preceding example, the comparisons shown in Table 5-5 would result. Thus the standard deviation of this regression would be calculated as .3705.

A far simpler approach is available using the data from the regression itself. If the standard deviation is 416.2, the variance is 416.2², or 173,222.44. The regression, as shown in the $r^2$ value, explains or accounts for .9999992 of all variations in the observed utilization. Therefore, only .0000008 is unexplained. The unexplained or chance variance is therefore .0000008 × 173,222.44 = .1386. (The slight difference between this figure and the .1373 previously calculated is due to rounding by the calculator, which can express only an $r^2$ to the nearest 7 decimal points.) The square root of .1385 = .3721. Although this is slightly different from the more thoroughly calculated version, it is enough to estimate precision. The precision of the regression should be roughly + 1.96 × $\dfrac{.3721}{1,358.6}$ = ± 0.05 percent, an extremely precise regression.

To repeat, the precision of a regression projection can be estimated as

$$\pm\ 1.96 \times \frac{\text{standard deviation of regression}}{\text{mean of observed utilization}}$$

for 95 percent confidence or

**Table 5-5** Comparisons of Predicted Values and Observation

| Independent | Predicted Dependent | Actual Observation | Difference | Difference² |
|---|---|---|---|---|
| 600 | 797.97 | 798 | 0.03 | .0009 |
| 800 | 1,064.02 | 1,064 | 0.02 | .0004 |
| 798 | 1,061.36 | 1,061 | 0.36 | .1296 |
| 1,064 | 1,415.20 | 1,415 | 0.20 | .0400 |
| 1,061 | 1,411.21 | 1.412 | 0.79 | .6241 |
| 1,415 | 1,882.12 | 1,882 | 0.12 | .0144 |
| 1,412 | 1,878.12 | 1,878 | 0.12 | .0144 |

$$.8238 \div (7 - 1) = .1373 \quad \sqrt{.1373} = .3705$$

$$1.645 \times \frac{\text{standard deviation of regression}}{\text{mean of observed utilization}}$$

below prediction for 95 percent confidence below the regression.

## SUMMARY

Autocorrelation differs from linear extrapolation in two ways. It bases its description of the past on relationships between pairs of observations rather than a full time series, and it projects the future based on the most recent relevant observation rather than on the entire time series. Like linear extrapolation, however, it can be done via graphic, mathematic or statistical analysis.

Graphic analysis of autocorrelation examines the relationship between a number of plotted pairs of utilization observations. All such relationships must be linear in the graphic mode. Graphics can be helpful in indicating whether an autocorrelation technique describes the past pattern or utilization well and whether a special form of autocorrelation such as time-lagging or unequal periods should be used. It is used more to select appropriate mathematic and statistical techniques than to describe actual forecasts.

Mathematic approaches to autocorrelation rely on identifying amounts or rates of change between early and later utilization observations. Such rates or ratios may be calculated on adjacent or time-lagged periods of equal or unequal length. The amounts or rates may be averaged, or if appropriate, subject to secondary analysis to develop the best possible pattern.

The statistical approach to autocorrelation is an autoregression. This technique enjoys the same advantages and disadvantages as the linear regression when applied to forecasting. Because it includes measures of past accuracy, however, it can be helpful in choosing alternative formulas and in explaining the choice to decision makers.

Chapter 6

# Analytic Methods

Linear extrapolation and autocorrelation methods for projecting utilization uncritically extend past patterns into the future. With the risk inherent in these methods recognized, a number of techniques carefully examine and systematically analyze past patterns before deciding how to project them into the future. These methods select one or more aspects of past patterns or give greater weight to some aspect as a basis for forecasting the future.

Three basic classes of analytic methods for projecting utilization are covered in this chapter:

1. moving averages
2. corrective weighting
3. time series analysis

Moving averages techniques systematically reduce the variability observed in past utilization in order to identify a basic underlying pattern that can be used to project the future. Corrective weighting techniques give greater weight to more recent experience while recognizing the overall pattern in past utilization. Time series analysis breaks down past utilization data into specific components, then employs each of the components to project the future.

## MOVING AVERAGES

The moving average approach to projecting future utilization is primarily designed to factor out wide fluctuations in past observations. It is suggested precisely when such fluctuations are present in past utilization data. By factoring out extreme fluctuations, moving averages facilitate detecting any underlying pattern. Once identified, this pattern can then be used to project future utilization.

The process is called *moving averages* because it calculates average utilization for multiple periods, moving ahead one period at a time. For example, if the data in Table 6-1 described utilization by month at an ambulatory surgery center:

The standard number of periods used in moving averages is either three or five. As indicated by Table 6-1, the more periods in the averages, the less fluctuation there tends to be among the averages. The actual observations vary from 150 to 350; three-month averages range from 210.0 to 296.7, less than half as much; five-month averages range from 224 to 268, about half as much as the three-month averages.

The forecast for the next period, i.e., the eleventh month in the preceding series, would be the moving average for the present month, i.e., 236.7 for three-month averages or 236.0 for the five-month version. Because moving averages are mean values of past observations, they are inherently conservative. Their projection of utilization can never be less or more than the lowest and highest observed values in past utilization.

The value of moving averages is their reduction of fluctuation. By examining moving averages, it is much easier to determine if there is any underlying trend. The preceding data, if analyzed via a linear regression, would produce widely different results comparing the raw data to the moving averages. The observations would yield a regression with a $r^2$ value of .001, which would project utilization of 244 for period 11. The three-year moving averages regression would have a $r^2$ value of .258 and project a utilization of 214.8 for period 11. The five-year regression would have a $r^2$ value of .429 and project 223.2 patients for period 11. By elimi-

**Table 6-1** Utilization by Month

| Month | Patient Surgeries | 3-Month Average | 5-Month Average |
|-------|-------------------|-----------------|-----------------|
| 1     | 150               |                 |                 |
| 2     | 300               |                 |                 |
| 3     | 240               | 230.0           |                 |
| 4     | 350               | 296.7           |                 |
| 5     | 180               | 256.7           | 244             |
| 6     | 270               | 266.7           | 268             |
| 7     | 200               | 216.7           | 248             |
| 8     | 160               | 210.0           | 232             |
| 9     | 310               | 223.3           | 224             |
| 10    | 240               | 236.7           | 236             |

nating fluctuations, the underlying pattern is more accurately identified. Whether this pattern proves effective in forecasting is of course another matter.

Where trends seem to be present in the moving averages, they may be used rather than the most recent average to project utilization. In the preceding illustration, there did seem to be somewhat of a trend present, though even with five-year averages the highest $r^2$ value obtained was still less than .500. Careful judgment should be used before relying on the trend to forecast utilization, as is true in any trend situation.

If the underlying trend seems likely to persevere *and* the pattern of fluctuations is a consistent and persistent one, a special modification of moving averages may be employed. This technique uses both trend and fluctuations to project future utilization. For example, if the data in Table 6-2 were observed:

A regression of the observations themselves yields a $r^2$ of .009 and a period 11 forecast of 274. A regression of the three-period averages yields a $r^2$ of .969 and a forecast of 290.2. The five-period regression would have a $r^2$ of .056 and a forecast of 277.5. The much higher $r^2$ value for the three-period average suggests that a repeating pattern of fluctuation is present, and is a three-period repeat.

This pattern can easily be observed by examination of the data in this illustration. Each three-year cycle goes through an increase of 200 followed by a drop of 100. The next cycle begins 10 or 20 surgeries ahead of where the prior cycle began and repeats the plus 200, minus 100 pattern. Thus the "eyeball estimate" for period 11 would be based on the expectation that it will be 200 more than period 10, i.e., 190 + 200 = 390.

This same pattern results mathematically if the moving average trend is used to forecast the next period's *moving average*. For example, if period 11 is to have a moving average of 290.2, then period 11 must be enough to

**Table 6-2** Future Utilization Projection

| Period | Utilization | 3-Period Average | 5-Period Average |
|--------|-------------|------------------|------------------|
| 1 | 150 | — | — |
| 2 | 350 | — | — |
| 3 | 250 | 250.0 | — |
| 4 | 170 | 256.7 | — |
| 5 | 370 | 263.3 | 258 |
| 6 | 270 | 270.0 | 282 |
| 7 | 180 | 273.3 | 248 |
| 8 | 380 | 276.7 | 274 |
| 9 | 280 | 280.0 | 296 |
| 10 | 190 | 283.3 | 260 |

raise the average of periods 9 and 10 to that level when combined with period 11. With an average of 290.2, the sum of periods 9, 10, and 11 must be 3 × 290.2, or 870.6. With periods 9 and 10 contributing 280 + 190 = 470, period 11 must contribute the difference, or 870.6 − 470 = 400.6. This would be the modified moving average projection for period 11 in contrast to the simple moving average projections of 283.3 (3-period) and 260 (5-period).

This simple moving average approach can be modified first by trending moving averages rather than projecting the most recent average as the forecast for next period. It can then be modified further, as described, to incorporate directly the pattern of fluctuations as well as the underlying trend. The decomposition of past patterns of utilization into trend and fluctuation is a form of time series analysis. Additional examples of this approach to forecasting are discussed later in this chapter.

## CORRECTIVE WEIGHTING

There are a host of specific approaches to correctively weighting past utilization experience as a basis for projecting future use of health services. The simplest approach is to weight each successive period's utilization in ascending order. Thus, if seven weeks of utilization of a clinic were chosen as a basis for forecasting, each period would be weighted from one to seven as in Table 6-3.

The unweighted average number of visits for this period would be 1,500 ÷ 7 = 214.3. By contrast the weighted average would be 6,400 ÷ 28 = 228.5. By giving greater weight to more recent experience, the trend of increasing utilization would be incorporated into the forecast of the next period's visits, i.e., 228.5. On the other hand such weighting is far more

**Table 6-3** Weighted Clinic Utilization

| Week | Visits | Week × Visits |
|------|--------|---------------|
| 1 | 150 | 150 |
| 2 | 200 | 400 |
| 3 | 250 | 750 |
| 4 | 180 | 720 |
| 5 | 210 | 1,050 |
| 6 | 240 | 1,440 |
| 7 | 270 | 1,890 |
| 28 | 1,500 | 6,400 |

conservative than a linear regression based on that trend. Such a regression would project use in the next period of 271.4 visits.

A second approach to weighting past utilization would be to weight the moving averages of the clinic's visits. Such an approach reduces the impact of wide variations from week to week, yet recognizes whatever trend might be underlying past experience. Using the same data as in the preceding unaveraged example results in the data shown in Table 6-4.

In this case the weighted moving average forecast for the next period would be 3,300 ÷ 15 = 220. This is less than the unaveraged forecast of 228.5 but still more than an unweighted average of all seven periods, which would forecast 1,500 ÷ 7 = 214.3. By giving some weight to more recent experience, some trend effect is incorporated into the forecast, but less than would be true with a trending technique per se. No weighting would produce a forecast in excess of what had already been experienced.

## EXPONENTIAL SMOOTHING

A more common adjustment technique called *exponential smoothing* is similar to autocorrelation in that it takes off from the most recent observation rather than the pattern of multiple past observations. It employs the difference between observed and expected utilization to generate a forecast of future utilization. Like the weighted moving average technique, it is also conservative in that it will not project a future beyond the range of the values used to analyze the past.

A standard notation for exponential smoothing is

$$F_{t+1} = \alpha\, O_t + (1 - \alpha)F_t$$

where

**Table 6-4** Moving Averages of Clinic Visits

| Week | Visits | Three-Week Moving Average | Weight | Weighted Average |
|------|--------|---------------------------|--------|------------------|
| 1 | 150 | | | |
| 2 | 200 | | | |
| 3 | 250 | 200 | 1 | 200 |
| 4 | 180 | 210 | 2 | 420 |
| 5 | 210 | 213.3 | 3 | 640 |
| 6 | 240 | 210 | 4 | 840 |
| 7 | 270 | 240 | 5 | 1,200 |
| | 1,500 | | 15 | 3,330 |

$F_t$   =  forecast for the present period
$O_t$   =  observed utilization for present period
$F_{t+1}$ =  forecast for next period
$\alpha$    =  weight between 0 and 1 reflecting degree of smoothing employed

To employ exponential smoothing, some technique must first be used to generate a forecast for the present period ($F_t$). A moving average technique might be used, for example. In the previous illustration the moving average for week 7 would have been the average of the three previous weeks, or 210. The observed utilization for period 7 was 190. Employing these values in exponential smoothing would yield the following:

$$F_8 = \alpha(190) + (1 - \alpha)\,(210)$$

With $\alpha$ taking any potential value from 0 to 1, the range of possible forecasts for period 8 is limited somewhere between 190 and 210. If $\alpha$ is given a weight of 1, $F_8$ becomes

$$1(190) + (1 - 1)(210) = 190$$

If $\alpha$ is given a weight of 0, $F_8$ becomes

$$0(190) + (1 - 0)(210) = 210$$

Should $\alpha$ be given a weight of 0.5, $F_8$ would be

$$.5(190) + (1 - .5)(210) = 95 + 105 = 200$$

The selection of a weight value for $\alpha$ is purely arbitrary, as for all smoothing techniques. The greater the weight given to $\alpha$, the greater is the credibility given to the most recent experience in contrast to whatever past experience was used to generate the forecast for the most recent period.

If an exponential smoothing approach had been used to generate a projection for period 7, that projection would be based on the following:

$$F_7 = \alpha O_6 + (1 - \alpha)F_6$$

If this is substituted into the formula for projecting period 8, the following expression results:

$$F_8 = \alpha(O_7) + (1 - \alpha)[\alpha O_6 + (1 - \alpha)F_6]$$
$$F_8 = \alpha(O_7) + \alpha O_6 + (1 - \alpha)F_6 - \alpha^2 O_6 - \alpha(1 - \alpha)F_6$$

which means that the $\alpha$ weight is squared when applied to the observed utilization in period 6. The use of an exponential weight in dealing with past observations results in the name exponential smoothing.

If there is no systematic pattern in past observations, the exponential smoothing produces forecasts similar to those of moving averages. The chief difference is the greater impact of the most recent period's experience. As shown, the maximum value possible as a forecast for period 8 would be 210 visits where a weighted moving average produced a forecast of 211.13. This is due to the fact that the most recent period showed 190 visits, thus pulling down the forecast for period 8.

If there is some sort of basic trend present in past observations, the exponential smoothing technique reflects it, but only partially. The higher the weight given to $\alpha$, the greater the extent to which the trend is reflected. In no case, however, can the forecast for the next period exceed the observed utilization of the present if the trend is upward, nor is the forecast below the present if the trend is downward. If there is confidence in the trend, one of the extrapolation techniques would be preferred. A smoothing technique is inherently conservative relative to past trends.

In order to give some cognizance to past trends but maintain some conservatism, an adjustment can be made to the exponential smoothing technique. Instead of using the forecast for the present period as a starting point, a forecast of the next period may be substituted as follows:

$$F_{t+1} = (F'_{t+1}) + \alpha(O_t - F_t)$$

A forecast for the next period, derived from moving averages, exponential smoothing, extrapolation, or some other technique, is used as the preliminary forecast $(F'_{t+1})$. The forecast for the present period, derived by the same technique used to develop $F_{t+1}$, is then compared to this forecast as a smoothing factor.

A series of observations as in Table 6-5 might warrant use of the modified exponential smoothing approach. The moving average forecast for period 8 would be 215.0. A simple exponential smoothing forecast for period 8 would be

$$F_8 = .5(225) + .5(203.3) = 112.5 + 101.65 = 214.15$$

A modified exponential forecast based on the moving average projection of 215.0 would be

**Table 6-5** Three-Period Moving Average

| Period | Visits | Three-Period Moving Average |
|--------|--------|------------------------------|
| 1 | 170 | |
| 2 | 185 | |
| 3 | 180 | 178.3 |
| 4 | 190 | 185.0 |
| 5 | 210 | 193.3 |
| 6 | 210 | 203.3 |
| 7 | 225 | 215.0 |

$$F_8 = F_8 + .5(O_7 - F_7) = 215 + .5(225 - 203.3) = 225.85$$

This modification enables the forecast to reflect past trends by factoring in the difference between past forecasts and observations. As can be seen by comparing the moving averages to actual observations, the smoothing techniques tend to fall behind trends, though they reflect them.

**TIME SERIES ANALYSIS**

Time series analysis, or *time series decomposition* as it is sometimes called, attempts to break down utilization experience into consistent and persistent components that are then separately used to forecast utilization for specific future periods. This analysis usually separates past experience into

- trend (directional variation)
- seasons (microcyclicity)
- cycles (macrocyclicity)
- error (unexplained variation)

A typical example of this analysis would examine yearly utilization of a hospital as containing some underlying trend from year to year and weekly and seasonal fluctuations within each year and cycle.

*Trends* in utilization over time can be identified through any of the techniques described in Chapter 4. Generally speaking, in time series analysis the preferred form for trend analysis is the simple linear regression. This technique has the advantage of specifically identifying how much of the change over time in utilization is explained by the trend, i.e., the $r^2$

value, and therefore how much remains to be explained by micro- and macrocycles or left in an error term.

*Microcycles* occur within the basic time unit examined. If the time unit is the year, then monthly utilization would be examined as a microcycle. If the time unit is a month or week, then day-of-the-week census or admission figures would represent microcycles. The purpose of the microcycle is to forecast utilization for a specific subunit of time once utilization for the basic time unit has been projected. Utilization for the basic unit is projected through some combination of trend and macrocycle.

*Macrocycles* describe variations around any linear trend describing utilization during basic time units. A trend in utilization of hospital care by month, for example, would be accompanied by a clear seasonal pattern of fluctuations. Utilization by day within each month would be affected by repeating day-of-the-week patterns. If the purpose of time series analysis were to predict utilization for a specific day of a specific month during this year, the within-the-year trend and seasonal macrocycle would be used to project the expected (average) daily census for the specified month. Day-of-the-week microcycle analysis would then project the expected census for a given day within the month.

If the task were to forecast utilization for a specific month next year, a trend and macrocycle could be used to project next year's average daily census. Then a seasonal or month-to-month microcycle would be used to project the average census or total patient days for the month. If desired, a further microcycle for daily census could then be used. If even more refined forecasts were desired, an hour-of-the-day microcycle might be employed.

Macrocycles can be identified from past data in a number of ways. As with all patterns of past utilization, an incremental approach moving from graphic through arithmetic to statistical analysis is recommended. Graphic analysis should indicate a number of useful facts regarding any apparent macrocycle.

- How many cycles are observed in past data?
- How frequently does the cycle repeat?
- Does it repeat with a constant or changing frequency?
- Is the cycle symmetrical—does it stray as far below the trend line as above it and spend the same length of time above as below?

### Illustration

The data cited in the discussion of a modified moving averages approach can be used to illustrate a cycle. These data would be portrayed graphically as in Figure 6-1.

**Figure 6-1** Macrocycle

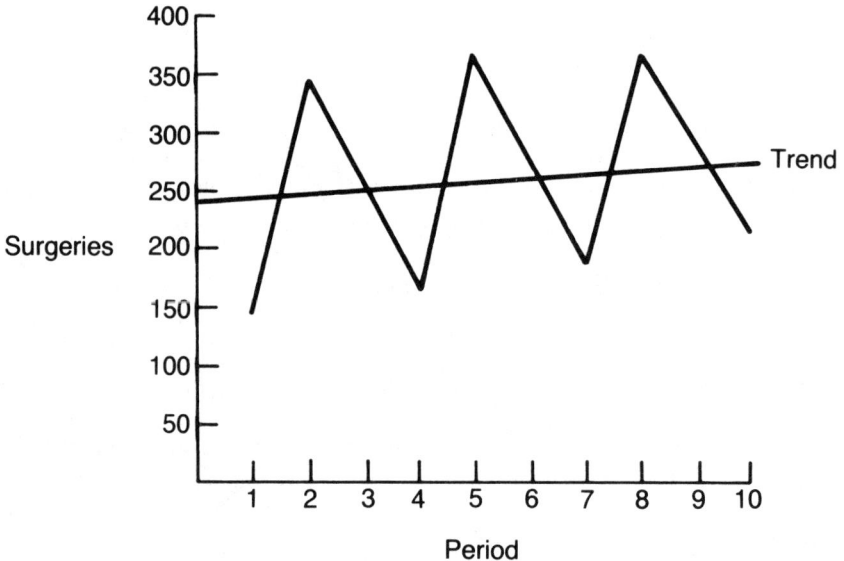

From this graphic analysis it appears that the macrocycle occurred three times, repeating every three periods consistently and with a symmetrical form. When the cycle is examined relative to the trend, it is clear that utilization varies roughly plus or minus 100 on either side of the underlying trend. With such neat, though atypical, data a forecast for the eleventh and twelfth periods could easily be derived without the use of even mathematical analysis.

Mathematical analysis would tend to refine the graphic portrayal of the pattern present in past utilization in most cases. In this illustration simple mathematics reveals that the cycle moves with the following sequence: +200, −100, −100, +200, −100, −100, etc. The trend moves forward with an underlying increase of 15 every three periods or 5 per period. If we had confidence in the persistence and consistency of both the trend and the cycle, we could forecast utilization as far into the future as we wished:

- Period 13 would be at the beginning of the fifth cycle. Thus, the trend of plus 5 per year should move utilization to 250 + (12 × 5) = 310 between period 1 and period 13. Because period 13 is the first period in its cycle, however, it should be 100 below its trend, or 310 − 100 = 210.

- Period 26 would be at the middle of the ninth cycle. By then the trend should have reached 250 + (25 × 5) = 375. Because the second period in a cycle is 100 above its trend, period 26 should have utilization of 375 + 100 = 475.

An arithmetic version of a microcycle can be expressed in terms of ratios of the expected, i.e., trend forecast value. Within any one year, for example, monthly utilization figures can be expressed as ratios to expected values. Within any week daily utilization can be expressed in terms of ratios to the weekly average. These ratios describe the relationships observed in the past. If such ratios have been fairly consistent and figure to persist they can be used to project future utilization over a microcycle period.

Days of the week often influence utilization. For inpatient hospital care, admissions tend to be fairly significant on Sunday, rise to a peak on Monday and Tuesday, then drop off toward Thursday and Friday with the low on Saturday. Daily inpatient census follows a similar pattern, with peak census midweek and the low on Saturday, but the census doesn't vary nearly as much as daily admissions within the week. Use of the hospital's emergency room tends to peak over the weekend, with Friday and Saturday nights particularly high.

Wherever sufficient experience is available, the relationship between the day of the week and the average for the week can be calculated. A set of ratios for daily admissions might look like the following:

| Sun. | Mon. | Tues. | Wed. | Thur. | Fri. | Sat. |
|------|------|-------|------|-------|------|------|
| 1.0  | 2.5  | 1.5   | 1.0  | 0.5   | 0.4  | 0.1  |

For any particular week, once the total admissions for the week have been forecast, daily admissions can be projected based on these ratios. If 70 admissions are expected during the week, the average would be 70 ÷ 7 = 10 per day. There should therefore be exactly 10 on Sunday, 25 on Monday, 15 on Tuesday, etc.

The ratios between day-of-the-week and weekly average have probably varied a little in the past. To reflect the inconsistency of past ratios, the standard deviation of these ratios should be calculated as well as their means. Consider the five weeks of experience in daily hospital admission ratios in Table 6-6, for example.

With these standard deviations it is possible to develop estimates of the *range* of admissions likely in a given week once the average for the week is forecast. If the average for the week is forecast as 12, for example, then Tuesday should be 1.5 × 12 = 18. With a standard deviation of 0.3, however, its one-standard deviation range would be ± 0.3 × 12 = ± 3.6.

**Table 6-6** Daily Hospital Admission Ratios

| Week | Sun. | Mon. | Tues. | Wed. | Thur. | Fri. | Sat. |
|---|---|---|---|---|---|---|---|
| 1 | 1.0 | 2.5 | 1.5 | 1.0 | 0.5 | 0.4 | 0.1 |
| 2 | 1.2 | 2.4 | 1.8 | 1.2 | 0.4 | 0.0 | 0.0 |
| 3 | 0.8 | 2.6 | 1.6 | 0.8 | 0.4 | 0.6 | 0.2 |
| 4 | 1.0 | 2.4 | 1.6 | 1.1 | 0.6 | 0.2 | 0.1 |
| 5 | 1.0 | 2.6 | 1.0 | 0.9 | 0.6 | 0.8 | 0.1 |
| Mean | 1.0 | 2.5 | 1.5 | 1.0 | 0.5 | 0.4 | 0.1 |
| Standard deviation | 0.14 | 0.1 | 0.3 | 0.16 | 0.1 | 0.32 | 0.07 |

Thus the chances are about two in three (68 percent) that Tuesday's admissions will be between $18 - 3.6 = 14.4$ and $18 + 3.6 = 21.6$. A two-standard deviation range would create a probability of 95 percent that it would include the actual Tuesday admission level. Unfortunately the range would be large, plus or minus 7.2, or 11 to 25.

Macrocycles may be described in a similar fashion if enough experience is available to analyze. Monthly variations during the year may be macrocycles if the forecast is intended to project utilization by month based on trend and variation during the year. If the macrocycle is one of trends and variations in annual utilization, the period of the cycle may be so long as to preclude detection. A cycle of 10 years may be possible to detect, but to get a clear picture of the consistency of past cycles, at least five cycles should be analyzed. This would mean that at least 50 years of data would be needed.

As indicated, a macrocycle can be calculated from only one cycle of experience. Employing such a cycle for forecasting is risky, however, because there is no basis for relying on its being both consistent and persistent.

## COMPUTER APPROACHES

Time series data may be analyzed through even more complex techniques. Box-Jenkins and Autoregressive Integrated Moving Averages (ARIMA) are two more commonly employed choices. It is impossible to describe the details of these techniques in this context. Moreover computer capability is essential in employing them. Sophisticated forecasting software packages should include these programs, however, where a more sophisticated time series analysis is desired.

The thing to keep in mind with any form of time series analysis is that like all projection techniques, it relies on the proper identification of past patterns and their persistence into the future. More complicated forms of analysis can succeed in identifying more complex patterns. No form of time series analysis can even guess as to the probable persistence of the patterns, however. An understanding of why patterns have occurred, together with reasoned confidence in their persistence, should be reached before any form of projection forecasting is used.

Analytic techniques, like projection techniques generally, should be used mainly in short-term forecasting. They are designed for use when the reasons for fluctuations in utilization patterns are unknown. Moving averages reduce the effect of fluctuations in forecasting, so this approach is designed for situations where the direction of fluctuations cannot be predicted. Corrective weighting is designed for situations where a trend in recent utilization deserves some recognition in estimating utilization in the next period.

Time series analysis is designed for use in situations where the total pattern of past utilization, its trend and fluctuations, is expected to continue. It is best employed in short-term forecasting unless there is great confidence that the entire pattern will continue for a long time. If some part of the pattern is expected to persist, e.g., the linear trend or one of the cycle patterns, that part may be employed to predict utilization while some other technique is used for other aspects of such utilization. A new trend might be forecast, for example, while the seasonal variation pattern is retained for predicting daily, weekly, or monthly fluctuations around that trend.

## SUMMARY

There are three basic categories of analytical approaches to projecting future use of health services. Moving average techniques combine utilization of previous periods in order to smooth wide variability, then forecast based on the underlying pattern. Corrective weighting gives greater weight to more recent experience, while constraining its projection of future use to be within the range of past experience. Time series analysis breaks down past utilization patterns into trend, cycles, and unexplained variations, then projects utilization in upcoming periods based on the total pattern of past use.

Like extrapolation and autocorrelation techniques, analytical approaches to forecasting can employ simple graphics, arithmetic, or statistical techniques to identify past patterns and project them into the future. The more complicated approaches require computer programs and voluminous data.

Even the most complex rely on the same basic logic, however: the extrapolation or projection of past utilization patterns into the future.

**Annotated Bibliography**

**Adam, G., et al.** "Forecasting Demand for Medical Supply Items Using Exponential and Adaptive Smoothing Models." In *Annual Proceedings of the American Institute for Decision Sciences,* p. 469. Atlanta: 1972.
    Describes use of smoothing techniques to forecast demand for specific items in central supply.

**Box, G., and Jenkins, G.** *Time Series Analysis: Forecasting Control.* San Francisco: Holden-Day, 1970.
    Describes time series techniques including what has come to be known as the Box-Jenkins computerized model.

**Brown, R.** *Smoothing, Forecasting and Prediction of Discrete Time Series.* Englewood Cliffs, N.J.: Prentice-Hall, 1963.
    Good general discussion of projection techniques.

**Harris, R., and Adam, E.** "Forecasting Patient Tray Census for Hospital Food Service." *Health Services Research* 10, no. 4 (Winter 1975): 384.
    Discusses superiority of an exponential smoothing technique in forecasting short-term inpatient utilization.

**Kao, E., and Tung, G.** "Forecasting Demand for Inpatient Services in a Large Public Health Delivery System." *Socio-Economic Planning Sciences* 14, no. 2 (1980); 97.
    Describes the Auto-Regressive Integrated Moving Average (ARIMA) technique of time series analysis for short-term forecasting of hospital utilization.

**Konnerman, P.** "Forecasting Production Demand in the Dietary Department." *Hospitals* 43 (September 1969): 102.
    Describes the use of a 10-week moving average technique to predict inpatient utilization in hospitals and resulting food demand.

**Sposato, D., and Spinner, A.** "Forecasting by a Modified Exponential Smoothing." *Health Services Research* 5, no. 2 (Summer 1970): 141.
    Describes the use of exponential smoothing to predict the number of insurance plan subscribers from year to year.

**Wood, S.** "Forecasting Patient Census—Commonalities in Time Series Models." *Health Services Research* 11, no. 2 (Summer 1976): 158.
    Describes use of ARIMA technique to forecast hospital census from one day to four weeks in advance.

# Chapter 7

# The Product Life Cycle

The concept of a *product life cycle* comes from marketing literature. It describes a pattern of sales of a product over time, beginning with its introduction and ending with its replacement by other products. The life-cycle pattern has a standard form but is subject to a number of variations. Care must be taken in applying the concept to health care, which is a service rather than a good and has its unique market characteristics. With appropriate care the concept can be helpful first in forecasting the probable pattern of utilization expected for a new program and second in forecasting specific levels of utilization over time.

## THE CONCEPT

The underlying concept in the product life cycle is that products pass through four basic phases when they are on the market. This period may be brief, as for pet rocks, diet shampoo (for fat-headed people), hula hoops, and other fad products. It may also be extremely long, as for food staples, the Model-T, or health care.

A *product* in marketing terms means a specific good or service that fills a specific need. If either the good or service or the need itself changes appreciably, a new product life cycle may begin. When baking soda became touted as a deodorant for refrigerators, for example, an old product began a new life cycle. Examples of distinct products in health care include specific technologies such as the CT scanner or yag laser; new ways of "packaging" or delivering services, such as outpatient surgery, walk-in medical clinics, or urgicenters; home health care; ways of paying for or organizing care such as health maintenance organizations (HMOs), preferred provider organizations (PPOs), cost-based reimbursement; as well as the basic categories of service: inpatient hospital care, surgery, nursing home care, etc.

The life-cycle concept suggests that each product passes through the following stages:

- development stage
- growth stage
- maturity stage
- aging stage

Portrayed graphically, the classic product life cycle is shown in Figure 7-1.

Essentially the stages represent first a period of slow growth. Any new innovation is presumed to require time to gain acceptance; hence initial sales are low and early growth slow. If the innovation is a successful one, it then reaches a stage of rapid growth, in which sales dramatically increase. The life-cycle concept recognizes that there is a limited market for any product and that sales always fall somewhat short of their theoretical full potential. At this point, growth slows and a plateau is reached. The concept also assumes that every product eventually dies, is replaced by something else, or at least declines markedly from its highest level of acceptance.

A good example of a product life cycle in the health care field is the CT scanner. Introduced in 1973, this new product experienced slow initial growth in sales from 1973 to 1975. Part of this was no doubt caused by certificate-of-need regulations, but part was also due to its new, unfamiliar, and changing technology. CT scanners experienced rapid growth in sales during the late 1970s and entered the maturing stage in the early 1980s.

**Figure 7-1** Classic Product Life Cycle

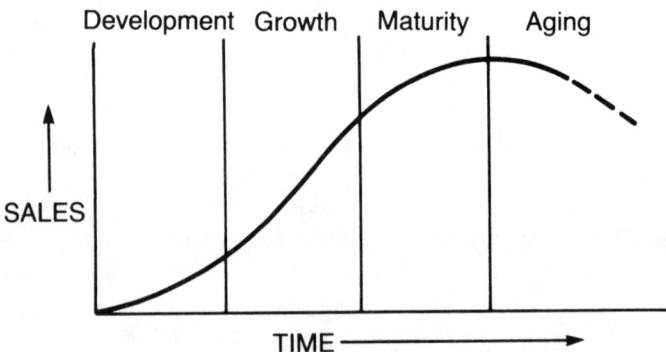

There are signs that sales will be pushed into the aging stage by nuclear magnetic resonance, positron emission tomography, or some other non-invasive diagnostic imaging device.

## VARIATIONS

The basic life-cycle concept tends to do well in describing or forecasting the basic pattern of growth in sales of an entire product in a market. Sales of specific *brands* may well follow a different pattern, however, depending on when they enter the market relative to the life cycle of the basic product. If a given product is the first one on the market, it may be the only available choice during the embryo stage. As such, it will follow the slow sales growth of the stage, as did the EMI scanner among CT scanners.

If other brands enter the market when the growth stage is reached, the first brand may never see dramatic growth. The newer brand may be technologically superior or have a stronger reputation or some other competitive distinction. If so, the initial brand may go right from development to aging and even disappear from the market. Under such circumstances its life cycle would look like Figure 7-2.

The brand that enters the market at the growth stage in the product's life cycle may not have to wait through slow early growth. If it can compete successfully and even competitively destroy the early brand, it may jump right into a rapid growth experience. On the other hand, other brands are likely to enter the market during the growth stage, and the second arrival

---

**Figure 7-2** Truncated Life Cycle

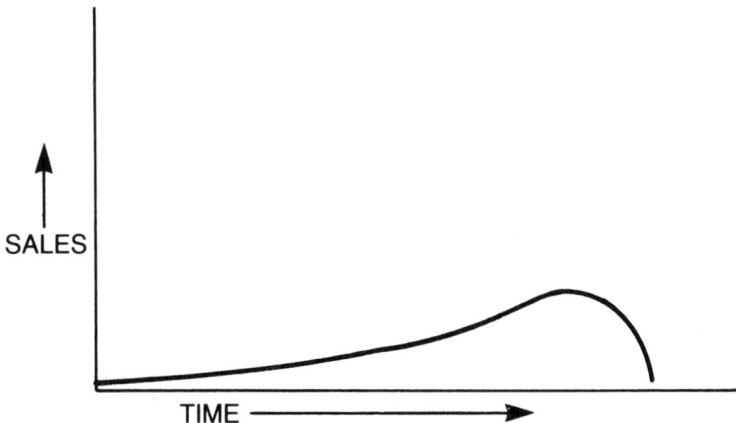

may find itself overtaken by these later arrivals. If so, its product life cycle may look like Figure 7-3.

If a brand enters the market during the maturity stage, it must compete for a share of the existing market because the market as a whole is not growing. If successful, it may experience the same rapid growth as if it entered during the growth stage. On the other hand there is less likelihood that it will experience additional new entries later. As a result, it is likely to be able to hold its market share longer. If so, its product life cycle would look like Figure 7-4.

Once the aging stage is reached, new brands are not entering the market, but the total demand for the product is dropping. The only way to hold sales levels long is to increase market share. This is extremely hard to do unless the brand develops a significant, new competitive distinction or competing brands voluntarily leave the market. In the long run sales drop and the life cycle ends.

**TRANSLATION TO HEALTH CARE**

To translate this basic concept into health care, we need only change the name *product* to *health service* or *program* and change the name *brand* to *provider*. As a service industry, the market for a given health care program is subject to specific geographic limits, as well. Walk-in clinics serve only people who live or work within a few miles. Ambulatory surgery programs, dialysis centers, and general hospitals can serve markets 25 to

**Figure 7-3** Second Arrival's Product Life Cycle

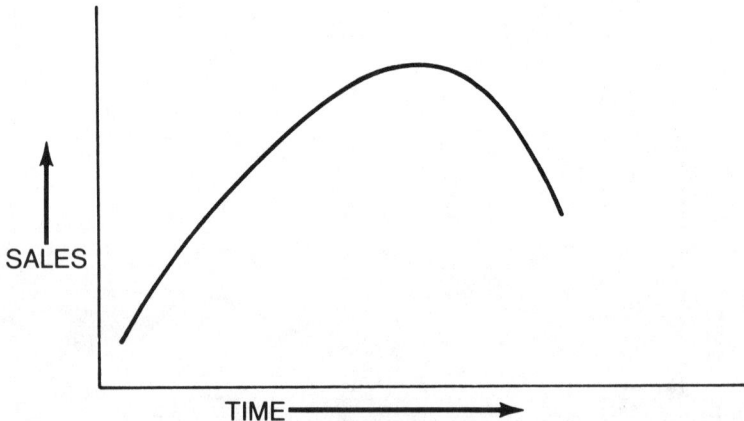

**Figure 7-4** Product Life Cycle After Maturity-Stage Entry

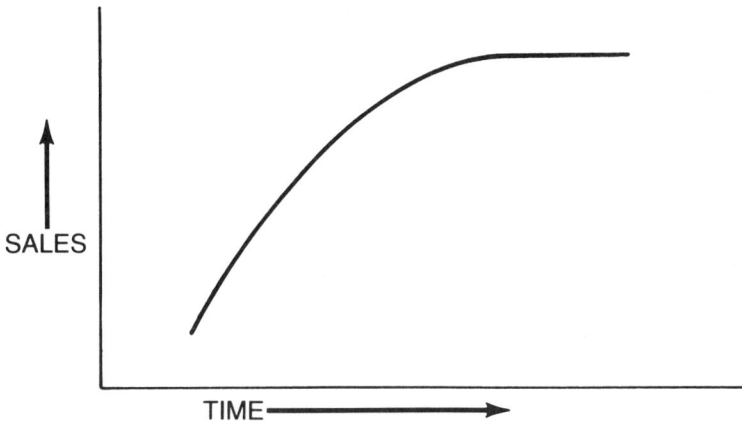

50 miles in radius. Highly specialized programs such as burn centers or open-heart surgery programs may serve markets ranging up to hundreds of miles.

The basic market for a product is not the same as for a specific provider. The geographic limits of the market for a specific service are determined by how far people could be expected to travel for such a service if only one provider were available. The markets for competing providers are influenced by the number and proximity of other providers, by physician and lay referral networks, and by specific linkages or barriers between providers and patients (e.g., HMO, PPO arrangements).

A basic health service such as inpatient care may have a life cycle of 100 years or so. It is likely, however, that it is in the aging stage. Outpatient surgery may be in the growth or maturity stage in different areas of the country. Nursing home care entered a dramatic growth stage as a result of Medicaid reimbursement and may be in another growth stage as the proportion of elderly increases dramatically before the early 21st century.

Specific providers may be at any number of different stages in specific service markets. The first walk-in clinic in the area was an innovator, but newer entries may have found better locations or used more effective marketing and be enjoying all the growth. With the present growth in physician supply, new providers entering the market for outpatient diagnostic and treatment services are probably inevitable in most areas.

Hospital emergency room (ER) utilization is probably a good illustration of the product life cycle applied to a specific health service. Originally emergency rooms served mainly emergencies as physicians handled routine care even after hours. As health insurance coverage for hospital emergency room care improved and the shortage of physicians let them limit their office hours, use of emergency rooms for routine care increased. Utilization of hospitals as sources of basic primary physician care grew dramatically during the 1960s and 1970s.

In the 1980s three factors are contributing to the plateauing and decline of ER volumes. First, insurance companies and government reimbursement programs are reducing their coverage for ER services. Second, private physicians are extending their office hours and making themselves more available to patients as their numbers increase and competition gets fierce. Third, walk-in clinics or urgicenters are offering the same convenience as ERs at lower cost. As a result, ER utilization figures take a nosedive.

## PRODUCT-LIFE-CYCLE FORECASTING

To employ the product-life-cycle concept in forecasting utilization of health services, it is first necessary to recall the basic principles embodied in the concept:

- New products tend to encounter slow acceptance at first.
- After early slow growth, a period of dramatic growth is likely *if the product is successful.*
- There is a limit to the market for any product, so growth will slow and stop.
- There's always a better product coming someday, so eventually demand for a product will diminish and possibly disappear.

With these basic principles in mind, the first thing to do in forecasting the use of a new program is to determine whether that program represents an innovation or simply a new brand, i.e., an additional provider entering a market already being served by one or more providers of the same services. The pure life-cycle pattern should be expected only to apply to truly new innovations, at least the first in the local market. One of the variations would be more likely to apply to new entries in markets already served by at least one other provider.

A new product or innovation must be perceived as new by the market in order for it to be expected to conform to the innovation adoption pattern of the product life cycle. A service that is technically new but is not perceived as different from what has been available won't qualify. Even an old program or one that is modestly changed may be perceived as new by the market, however, and follow the pattern well. The baking soda used to deodorize refrigerators is probably the best example of this principle.

A product must also be new to the specific market that exists for that product. That market is the set of people or organizations that could decide to buy the product or use the service. Hospitals were the initial markets for CT scanners, though physician groups have come in as well. Physicians are the market for using most inpatient services and specific technologies in most cases. Patients are the market for urgicenters and may influence the use of ambulatory surgery. Families are the principal market for nursing homes, though social agencies and churches may influence market choices as well. Services or programs that are new to those who decide whether and where to seek care should be classed as innovations.

The shape of the pattern of "sales" in the basic product life cycle is that of an ogive. It is essentially a cumulative distribution, such as that of the total number of patients being treated in the first-ever dialysis program or the first CT scanner. It can also apply to the total utilization of a new service in a total market, such as the use of dialysis in the United States over time or the use of CT scanners nationwide. To use the ogive in forecasting, it is necessary to establish a starting point and estimate the pattern of growth in utilization over time.

A common practice in marketing circles is to employ the normal statistical distribution as the mathematical model for the innovation adoption curve, the first three phases of the product life cycle. This model views the total market (physicians, patients, employers, hospitals, depending on what the product is) as capable of being broken up into six groups:

1. innovators
2. early adopters
3. early majority
4. late majority
5. laggards
6. holdouts

These six categories are applied to the normal statistical distribution in Figure 7-5.

According to this model 2½ percent of the market are innovators, the first to adopt a new product, to use a new service. These could be the first physicians to use a new drug, the first surgeons to try outpatient surgery, the first patients to come to an urgicenter, or the first hospitals to buy a CT scanner, for example. Sociologists would characterize these innovators as social isolates, however, not the leaders of their group. They tend to

**Figure 7-5** Market Distribution

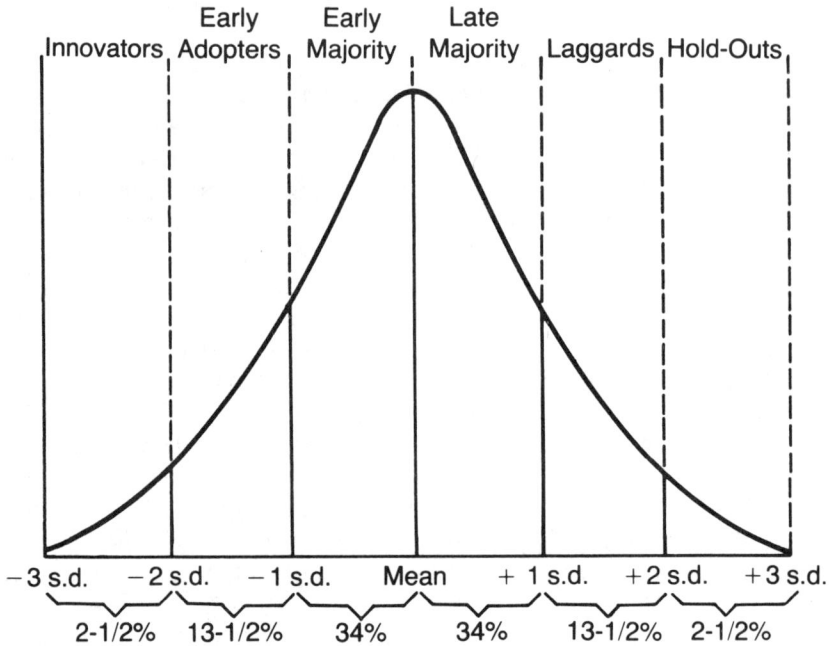

try new things because they are new. As such, they have little influence on others because they are not seen as reflecting the values of their peers but rather as somewhat radical and flighty. With the normal distribution, they are seen as a group that is more than two standard deviations from the mean in terms of similarity to the group and therefore covers only 2½ percent of the whole.

Early adopters are a little different from the average in that they try things early, though not first. They make up their minds quickly and are open to new ideas, but they don't jump at the first new thing just because it is new. These are the people who are between one and two standard deviations from the mean and include 13½ percent of the population. The early and late majority groups differ only slightly from the mean and from each other. Early majority members are more in contact with the early adopters, hence learn about innovations a little quicker and are slightly more willing to change. With 34 percent in each group, the early and late majority together make up over two-thirds of the total, 68 percent.

The laggards are slow to change and tend to take a wait-and-see, show-me attitude toward anything new. They wait to be swayed by the sheer numbers of their peers who have changed their behavior and take a conservative length of time to be convinced. They constitute the same proportion of the population as the early adopters, 13½ percent.

The holdouts are social isolates just as the innovators. Their response to new innovations is to resist change like the plague. They not only don't use electric razors, they probably still use a straight razor and a shaving brush. They tend to be older and stuck in their ways. They may never adopt the new product, but if they do, they add little to total utilization anyway as they represent only 2½ percent of the population or market.

If the normal distribution is portrayed in a cumulative fashion and if it is applied along time rather than across the market, it becomes the innovation adoption curve ogive (Figure 7-6). The key to using this ogive in forecasting is to estimate or measure some parameters of the curve and project the rest from these. If the total market size is known, for example, the forecasting task may be to estimate how soon each step of the adoption process occurs so as to estimate when saturation is reached. If the size of the market is not known, the forecasting task may be to fit early experience to the curve as a basis for estimating where the curve ends.

To employ the normal distribution ogive in forecasting utilization of a new program, the challenge is to fit initial utilization figures to the curve.

**Figure 7-6** Innovation Curve Ogive

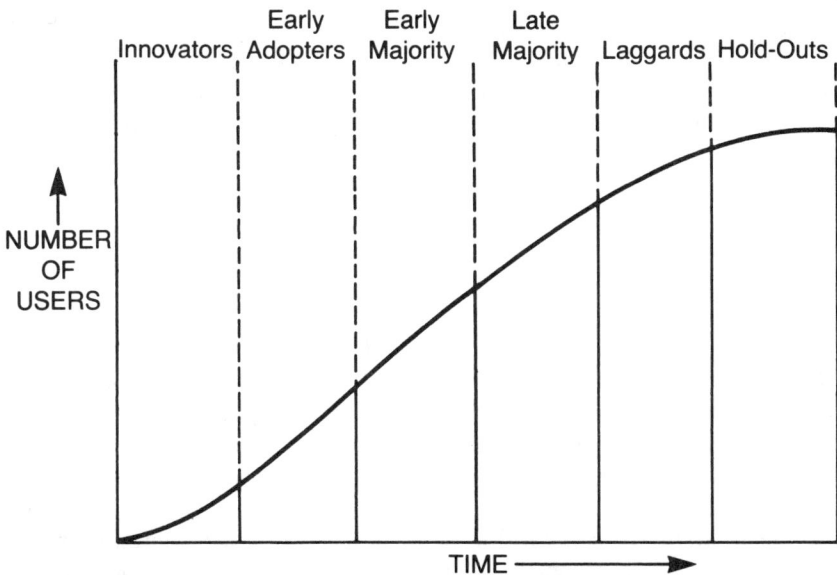

For example, if there were 25 registrants to a new program during the first month of operation of a new clinic, then 135 during the second month, this would fit the pattern well. If the first month's registrants are thought of as the innovators, they represent 2.5 percent of the total market. If so, the total market is 25 ÷ .025 = 1,000. By the same token, if the second month's registrants are treated as the early adopters, they should comprise 13.5 percent of the total. If so, the total will be 135 ÷ .135 = 1,000. That these two estimates of the total market agree is a strong indication that the pattern fits.

The more utilization experience available to analyze, of course, the more likely the correct pattern will be identified. If the third month's registrants amount to 340, that would strongly ratify the previous projection. Because the early majority is supposed to represent 34 percent of the total and 340 ÷ .34 = 1,000, the third month's experience yields the same result as the previous two. On the other hand, if a projection of growth must be made earlier, the forecast may not be able to wait until the expected pattern is strongly confirmed.

In practice, initial utilization does not fit the expected pattern as perfectly as in this illustration. If the first month's registrants amount to 25, the second month's registrants may be 200 or 500 or any number other than 350. On the other hand it is rarely necessary to project the timing or extent of growth of a new program with 100 percent accuracy. Developing a rough estimate of these two parameters is all that would be needed in most cases.

If the first month's registrants are 25 and the second month's 270, for example, each produces a different projection for the total. The first month would project 25 ÷ .025 = 1,000 and an expected growth pattern of 25, then 135, then 340, then 340, then 135, then 25. The second month would project 270 ÷ .135 = 2,000 and an expected growth pattern of 270, 680, 680, 270, and 50. The two together suggest that total registrants will amount to something between 1,000 and 2,000.

In order to project next period's growth, total utilization expected, or whatever parameter of utilization is to be forecast, it is first necessary to determine what *period* is logical for use in the model. In the preceding example the first two months suggest that a month fits well enough. Had the first month's utilization totaled 25 and the second month 50, a guess might be made that a longer period of adoption was likely or else the model doesn't fit. Had initial utilization been 25 and the next month's 600, the possibility exists that a shorter period was at work or that the model doesn't fit.

Some periods are a natural phenomenon based on the nature of the market. A year is a natural period for a number of market choices, for example. Purchases of major equipment are budgeted annually, so sales of CT scanners would naturally follow an annual pattern. Selection of an HMO option by employees also occurs only once a year for each employee group; hence HMO growth may follow a yearly period pattern where it is truly an innovation.

Other market choices may be monthly. If purchases of smaller items are discussed and approved at monthly meetings, for example, then one-month periods will probably work. If families plan elective use of health services based on monthly paychecks or if ads for the service appear once a month, then a one-month period may apply as well. The only way to select the proper period is to understand the dynamics of the market. Hence, although the innovation adoption curve is a naive projection technique by definition, it requires that choices be made on the basis of good judgment in order to be used.

Table 7-1 shows examples of cumulative distribution levels taken from the normal distribution. In each case the less the relative increase from one period to the next, the more periods there are in the pattern, hence the slower the growth expected.

As indicated by these data, in a 24-period situation, each period during the initial growth stage is less than twice as great as the previous period, rather is roughly half again as great. In a 16-period situation early utilization would roughly double each period. In a 12-period situation initial growth is over three times per period, but growth slows quickly. In a 6-period situation the second period is more than 4 times as great as the first, but the third is only 2½ times the second, showing both faster growth and faster maturing.

In addition to the normal distribution there are literally an infinite number of alternatives for projecting early utilization levels in the form of a logistic curve. If the size of the total potential market is known, i.e., if there is a known limit to the number of potential users of a program, it becomes relatively simple to translate initial utilization levels and the known limit into the expected growth pattern. Most statistical software packages execute the necessary analysis to produce the best choice of growth curves.

Like all curve-fitting projection techniques, an innovation adoption curve relies on proper identification of the pattern in utilization experienced. A logistic curve in the form of a log-linear regression (Chapter 4) offers the $r^2$ value as a measure of the goodness of fit. The arithmetic alternative is to apply a curve to succeeding periods of utilization to see if they individually and collectively yield roughly the same result, as illustrated in previous discussion.

**Table 7-1** Cumulative Distribution Levels

| Users | | | | | Period | | | | | |
|---|---|---|---|---|---|---|---|---|---|---|
| | 1 | 2 | 3 | 4 | 5 | 6 | 7 | 8 | 9 | 10 |
| *24 Periods* | | | | | | | | | | |
| New users | 5 | 7 | 10 | 16 | 26 | 37 | 58 | 82 | 112 | 146 |
| Total users | 5 | 12 | 22 | 38 | 64 | 103 | 161 | 243 | 355 | 501 |
| *16 Periods* | | | | | | | | | | |
| New users | 9 | 19 | 37 | 73 | 132 | 220 | 330 | 450 | 450 | 330 |
| Total users | 9 | 28 | 65 | 138 | 270 | 490 | 820 | 1,270 | 1,720 | 2,050 |
| *12 Periods* | | | | | | | | | | |
| New users | 12 | 41 | 125 | 238 | 446 | 740 | 740 | 446 | 238 | 125 |
| Total users | 12 | 59 | 166 | 404 | 850 | 1,590 | 2,330 | 2,776 | 3,014 | 3,139 |
| *6 Periods* | | | | | | | | | | |
| New users | 25 | 135 | 340 | 340 | 135 | 25 | | | | |
| Total users | 25 | 160 | 500 | 840 | 975 | 1,000 | | | | |

Like all projection techniques, however, the innovation adoption curve relies on the persistence of past patterns. If a competing program opens in the same market, it may cut off growth abruptly and truncate the expected pattern. Similarly a major publicity or advertising campaign may create a new spurt of growth after early returns show only gradual increases in utilization or even decline. The innovation adoption curve is likely to fit best when no major developments in the market disrupt the "natural" diffusion of new behavior within the market.

## SUMMARY

The product-life-cycle model represents a way of using utilization data from a period early in the history of a new service to project subsequent utilization. It is a special form of time series analysis based on past experience with innovative products entering the market. Although it is ideally suited to the projection of the sales of products, it can be applied to the projection of the use of services.

The concept must be translated both conceptually and mathematically into health services terms in order to be useful. Although a host of logistic or innovation adoption curves may be tried on past utilization data to see which fits best, the normal distribution model represents a commonly applied choice. If early utilization experience can be made to fit this or any other model, it can be used to predict both the rate of growth in use of a new service and the ultimate total utilization such a service can reasonably expect.

**Annotated Bibliography**

**Coleman, J., et al.** "The Diffusion of an Innovation among Physicians." *Sociometry* 20 (1957): 253.

Describes a sociometric approach to identifying innovators, early adopters, etc., among physicians.

**Heeler, R., and Husted, T.** "Problems in Predicting New Product Growth for Consumer Durables." *Management Science* 26, no. 10 (October 1980): 1007.

Describes the use of the product-life-cycle concept to predict sales of expensive consumer goods.

**Mahajan, V., and Muller, E.** "Innovation Diffusion and New Product Growth Models in Marketing." *Journal of Marketing* 43, no. 4 (Fall 1979): 55.

Discusses the innovation adoption and product-life-cycle curves as they can be applied to predicting market growth.

**Tigert, D., and Farivar, B.** "The Bass New Product Growth Model: A Sensitivity Analysis for a High Technology Product." *Journal of Marketing* 45, no. 4 (Fall 1981): 81.

Describes the use of a specific type of innovation adoption curve in predicting the adoption of complex technologies similar to the types used in delivering health services.

**Venkatesan, M., et al.** "HMOs: Product Life Cycle Approach." *Health Care Management Review* 5, no. 2 (Spring 1980): 59.

Discusses the possibility of using the product-life-cycle model to forecast the growth of HMO enrollment.

# Part III

# Prediction Techniques

Where projection techniques treat future utilization as a function of averages, trends, or other patterns in past utilization, prediction techniques treat future utilization as a function of the present or future status of some other factors. The utilization of health services to be forecast is *predicated* on one or more other variables. In research terms utilization is a *dependent variable* to be forecast as a function of one or more *independent variables*.

There is a basic, though often unstated, assumption made in all prediction techniques that there is some logical cause-and-effect link between independent and dependent variables. A selected independent variable or predictive factor may not *cause* utilization in the usual sense, but at least it is presumed to be linked to use of health services in some causal dynamics system. Thus, if there is a predicted or experienced change in an independent variable, there is reason to expect a related change in the dependent variable.

If use of health services were treated as a function of almost any variable, there is some likelihood that a strong mathematical association can be found. If only one or a few observations are analyzed, it is possible to calculate the association or mathematical relationship between use of health services and almost anything that can be counted and varies over time: sun spots, automobile sales, newspaper circulation. The concern must be that some associations might be spurious, that is, the result of chance rather than a true relationship. Spurious associations would not be expected to have any predictive value.

Chapter 8 discusses the causal context for prediction, the dynamics known to affect the utilization of health services. A number of causal models are discussed as having potential value in helping us to understand why utilization occurs and how to use that understanding to predict changes in utilization. The types of causal factors identified through research studies as being strongly linked to use of health services are identified and examined for predictive value.

Chapter 9 covers the most important causal factor in terms of utilization of health services: the population that will use them. The size of the service population or market for health services, its demographic characteristics, and other population factors are analyzed in terms of their predictive value. Techniques for identifying the probable impact of specific population factors treated one at a time are examined. A critical concern relative to one of the most useful demographic characteristics of a population, its age, is also discussed.

Chapter 10 examines environmental factors that can be used to predict utilization of health services. Included in such factors are aspects of the environment that a provider organization may be able to control or at least influence, hence determine rather than merely forecast the future. In such cases what is predicted is actually the expected consequences of a provider's intervention on health services utilization. Also included are factors that, like demographic features of the population, can usually only be forecast by a provider rather than controlled or influenced.

Chapter 11 discusses ways to predict the consequences of multiple factors acting simultaneously on health services utilization. The sorts of multiple-variable or multivariate techniques available may require use of computers in many cases but many can be handled on modern handheld calculators. The use of multivariate techniques carries with it some new risks as well as new possibilities in forecasting, both of which should be identified and appreciated as part of selecting and employing any specific technique.

Prediction techniques are, generally speaking, more complex but more reliable than projections. If a good predictive variable can be identified, if its relationship to health services utilization can be accurately measured, if its present or future status can be accurately determined, and if its relationship to use of health care persists in essentially the same form, prediction tends to produce better forecasts than projection. Prediction techniques can be used in intermediate and even long-range forecasting, for example, where projection is not recommended for more than immediate-range forecasts.

The general risk in prediction, aside from the technical uncertainties of specific techniques, is treating it as objective and scientific because it employs quantitative analytical tools. At the base of any prediction is a great reliance on human judgment, however. The selection of what predictive factors to use is purely a matter of choice. The decision as to what mathematical relationship to use in making a prediction is also purely a judgment call. Once judgments are made, prediction techniques produce forecasts based entirely on objective, quantitative analysis, but this does not escape the necessity for relying on human judgment in the first place.

Also, like projection, prediction relies on perseverance or persistence. Where projection relies on the persistence of past patterns in utilization itself, prediction relies on the perpetuation of whatever relationship between utilization and some independent variables is used to predict the future. Thus, like all forecasting, prediction ultimately calls for a confident belief that the past can be relied on as a basis for estimating the future.

In addition prediction calls for confidence that the relationship between the independent variables and health services utilization has been accurately identified. Moreover it requires faith in the accuracy of any forecast of the independent variables used to predict the dependent, unless time lagging is used, in which case the only belief required is that the present state of the independent variables has been accurately measured.

In spite of the added items of faith required in prediction, forecasts based on predictive relationships usually do turn out better than those based only on observed patterns in past utilization. Moreover, if predictions prove inaccurate, there is greater likelihood that the reasons can be identified because causal dynamics have been addressed. Thus, the use of prediction can benefit from organizational learning and experience over time where projection offers only simplicity of application.

# Chapter 8

# Causal Context

To predict utilization of health services as a function of some other factors, some appreciation for the causal context in which utilization occurs is useful, if not essential. To link a forecast of utilization to a decision requires that part of that causal context be established, namely, the consequences of utilization, its impact on success criteria of the organization. To forecast utilization by any technique, it is advisable to identify the rest of the causal context, the preceding dynamics that lead to utilization. To use a prediction technique, some understanding of the precedent dynamics is needed if only to select proper independent variables on which future utilization is dependent.

We are fortunate in having access to a vast body of literature on the causal context for utilization of health services and on specific factors thought to be linked to such utilization. Numerous causal models have been suggested as useful in explaining why and predicting to what extent people use health services. Hundreds of articles have been written linking utilization to one or more measurable aspects of people, their environment, or the health system itself.

Without specifying exactly how various factors relate to each other, a basic model can be described; it at least identifies categories of factors known to have some sort of causal relationship to use of health services. One set of categories relates to the users of health services and their social, psychological, and behavioral characteristics. Another set relates to the providers of, payers for, and regulators of health services, which go together to make up the health care system. A third set covers the environment in which all function. All categories tend to relate to all others, so the model, even simply expressed, is a fairly complex one.

## PEOPLE FACTORS

Characteristics of the users of health services known to affect their use fall into three basic categories: demographic factors, psychographic fac-

101

tors, and behavioral factors. Demographics cover the factual, objective attributes of users, their family, and cultural contexts, the sorts of characteristics listed in census data. Psychographics cover subjective attributes, the content of people's minds, both of users of health services and their family–cultural context. Behavioral factors include all behavior that impacts on health status, as well as behaviors related to use of services.

## Demographics

Demographic characteristics of user populations include a vast array of attributes that can be used to describe people. Among the most important are numbers of people, their age mix, health status, ethnicity, income, education, whether covered by health insurance, gender mix, and place of residence. Demographic factors have great advantages as predictors of health service use. They are objective, readily measurable, and often available in population forecasts developed by outside experts. They have two great disadvantages as well. They are only partially discriminatory in explaining specific preferences among competing providers, and they are rarely if ever subject to influence by the forecasting organization.

*Numbers* of people in the population represent the most readily available and useful demographic factor. With census data available down to census tract, block, and block face, the numbers of people residing in a service area can usually be counted with great accuracy. Moreover, with many commercial as well as governmental organizations having great interest in future population levels, good forecasts of population numbers are likely available, even for long-term forecasting. As forecasts, they are always risky but are likely to be among the most accurate of all demographic factors forecast.

*Age mix* is perhaps second only to numbers in terms of being an important determinant of health care use and both readily available for present populations and well forecast for the future. Some services are virtually total functions of age: pediatric services use is by definition limited to an age group; obstetrics is generally limited to women in a specific age segment. Other services are greatly influenced by age mix; inpatient hospital use is over four times higher in the over-65 age group than the under-65; use of nursing homes by age group is almost restricted to the over-65 segment and increases dramatically in the over-75 and over-85 groups.

*Health status* may seem too obvious a demographic characteristic to mention as related to health service use. There is certainly no surprise in findings that people who are ill use health care more than those who are healthy. People with specific conditions, including chronic disease and disability, can be predicted to use specific types and even precise numbers of services, e.g., kidney dialysis patients. The drawback to use of health status characteristics in forecasting is the difficulty of getting either accurate measures of current health status or *any* forecast of future status.

*Ethnicity* can be related to use of health services in a number of ways. Some ethnic groups are culturally isolated from the health care system and manifest low use of most services or use specific subsystems such as Indian Health Service clinics and hospitals. Others may prefer or be forced to use only specific providers such as Chinatown Hospital in San Francisco, Jewish hospitals serving kosher food for orthodox Jews, or public hospitals and clinics for ethnic groups not feeling welcome at private sources of care. Ethnic mix is hard to measure and often difficult to predict. Who would have predicted in 1970 the numbers of Indochinese refugees living in the United States by 1980? Who knows what refugee group might arrive during the 1980s?

*Income* and *education* tend to be highly correlated with each other and linked to differential use of health care. People with higher educations tend to use more preventive services, for example, and those with higher incomes can afford to use more elective services such as plastic surgery. Use of physician services tends to increase with higher education and income, for example. Income and education data are available from census information about present populations. They tend not to change much over time, however, or not be subject to accurate forecasting if they do.

Whether people are covered by *health insurance* and whether their coverage includes deductibles or co-insurance or covers fully, partially, or excludes specific services are important factors relative to their use of health services. Those covered by health insurance, especially those with first-dollar or full coverage, tend to use significantly more high-cost care such as hospital inpatient care, surgery, etc., than those less well covered. Deductibles and copayment requirements have been shown to reduce utilization compared to full coverage. Moreover, being covered versus not covered strongly influences where people go for care because it influences where they will be welcomed. The drawback with respect to health insurance coverage is that it is not fully measured in the kind of detail most useful in predicting use of health services and not readily forecast as a characteristic of a service population.

*Gender mix* is a strong factor in use of health services generally, as well as a determinant of some kinds of service use such as obstetric care and gynecological services. Women are much more likely to be found in nursing homes, for example, though this has more to do with their outliving their husbands than with gender-related health status. Women tend to be slightly lower users of health services in younger years, especially of care related to violence and accidents, then use slightly more care as they grow older. On the other hand gender mix changes little over time, hence often produces no influence in forecasts.

*Residence* is an influential demographic factor in both general and specific terms. Residents of rural versus suburban versus urban areas tend to use care at different rates, though income and occupation are greatly involved in some differences. Moreover, residents of some areas of the country, even some counties versus others in the same state, use care differently. This may be due somewhat to health system differences, what McClure calls the difference between conservative and aggressive medical practice. For whatever reason, where people live makes a great deal of difference to use of health care. In forecasting, the challenge is to decide whether this is a permanent or temporary phenomenon, linked to the population itself or to the providers serving that population.

In addition to these factors *occupation* patterns can greatly influence health service use. Some jobs are simply more hazardous than others: mining, forestry, fishing, and agriculture have special risks of injury while executives suffer from stress-related conditions. Working in shipyards accounted for asbestos-caused lung disease, coal mines are linked to black lung and cotton mills to brown lung disease. In addition to links between occupation and disease or injury, some work places offer health services and can produce positive effects on health through prevention and promotion. For forecasting purposes, only *changes* in occupational mix or work-place health programs need be considered in most cases.

Any demographic factors that affect population size, age mix, gender mix, income, education, ethnicity, residence, health status, occupation, or health insurance are also potentially important, at least indirectly, in forecasting use of health services. All the demographic factors mentioned are likely to be linked to each other, like age and income, age and health status, health status and income. Retired people tend to have lower incomes, as do young people beginning careers. Older people acquire more chronic disease, while young people, especially males, are more at risk for quadriplegia, for example. People too ill or disabled to work have lower incomes as a consequence.

The interaction among such independent variables complicates their use in forecasting utilization of health services by any population. In most cases the key is to select one or more factors because they are strongly and consistently linked to health service use, can be measured accurately and forecast reliably, and are subject to enough change to make a difference. (See discussion of change factors in Chapter 13.) The factors most strongly linked, most reliably forecast, and most significantly changing have the greatest impact on future utilization, hence are the most important to consider in developing a forecast.

**Psychographics**

Psychographic factors are subjective characteristics of populations covering what people know, believe, and feel about things. Factors include what people know, believe, and feel about themselves and their health, about health services and the health system, and about specific providers of service. Psychographic factors are far better discriminators of who will use specific sources of care than are demographic factors. Moreover they are far more readily influenced by provider organizations than are demographics. On the minus side they are almost never forecast objectively by outside agencies.

*Health status* beliefs, one's perceived health status and perceptions of the health status of others, have a great deal to do with whether people seek care, where, and when. Perceived emergencies tend to be followed by emergency care pursuit, even if no "true" emergency is present. Ignorance as to the meaning of symptoms may lead to delay in seeking treatment. Embarrassment over unmarried pregnancy and fear of it becoming known by others may explain some of the delay in seeking prenatal care common to teenage pregnancies, for example. One's perception of health status is certainly influenced by actual health status, but both denial of real problems and perception of nonexistent ones are commonplace.

Perceptions as to the efficacy versus pain, discomfort, or indignity attending *health services* are also major influencers of health care use. Much is being done, for example, to change the image of dental care as a painful process. The CT scanner provides an excellent example of a painless replacement for painful and risky alternatives such as angiography and pneumoencephalography. Hospitals are even using satisfaction-guaranteed-or-your-money-back approaches to improving their images as sources of bad food and impersonal treatment. A constant challenge in health care is to convince people of the effectiveness of specific services without promising results, thereby being open to suit for breach of contract.

People tend to differ widely in their perceptions and knowledge of the health care delivery system. Some have a good working knowledge of how to obtain needed care, select their own specialists, and "shop" for the best-known or best-reputation providers. Others are relatively uninformed about access to the system and simply seek the most readily available provider. A few feel isolated from the system and rarely use it at all, unless emergencies arise. Social, cultural, economic, and ethnic factors are likely to be linked to perception differences, but it is the perceptions themselves that affect use of health services.

In addition to variations in the overall impressions and knowledge that people have of the health system, there are wide differences in perceptions of specific providers. Thoughts on the preferability of specialists versus generalists for specific problems; for surgeons or internists; for chiropractors, podiatrists, or acupuncturists versus allopathic and osteopathic physicians vary widely. Preferences for male versus female physicians; younger versus older practitioners; solo practitioners or group practices; antiseptic, clinical surroundings or warm, homelike environments also vary greatly. To forecast selection of specific classes of providers or individuals, it is necessary to appreciate psychographic preferences. The role of marketing is to design provider features that conform to such preferences, then communicate persuasively about them.

**Behavior**

The use of any specific health service is a specific behavior, but it is influenced by other behaviors, including the use of other health services. Almost all behavior potentially affects health service use if it affects health status. Thus smoking, drinking, use of drugs, diet, exercise, employment, and everything that makes up life style, affects health service use at least indirectly. It has been shown in a number of studies that the use of mental health services tends to reduce the use of physical health services. The use of preventive services is supposed to reduce use of curative services; early detection can at least reduce the intensity of subsequent use of curative and rehabilitative care.

Many health services are intended to substitute for each other. Ambulatory surgery replaces inpatient use; home health care keeps people out of institutions. Going to a nurse-midwife can replace or at least reduce the use of an obstetrician's services; alternative birthing centers and home delivery replace use of obstetric care in hospitals. Thus much of the job of forecasting health services use reflects anticipated changes in the use of related and alternative health services.

Like psychographics, behavior is susceptible to influence and even control by the health service provider. The extent to which people comply with advice is a field of its own, with many characteristics of providers and their interactions with patients playing an important role. Hospital inpatients are largely under the control of their physicians when it comes to their use of health services, though permission must be obtained for surgery, and many patients do leave the hospital against medical advice.

Much health-related behavior is presumably related to psychographics. People's attitude toward and preferences among health services and alternative providers may be changed with the expectation that their subsequent behavior will be changed. Program features can be designed to make them more attractive to potential users, or persuasive communication may be able to alter attitudes by adding information to people's consideration or changing their image of health services and providers. Personal selling, publicity, and advertising may be used to alter behavior by modifying attitudes.

Behavior may be approached more directly by simply facilitating a desired behavior. Making services more readily available may increase their use without relying on a change in attitude. Using mobile screening services for diabetes or hypertension, for example, may greatly expand their use with no discernible change in popular attitudes toward such services. Improving access to care can simply facilitate the translation of preference into purchase by individual patients. Positive attitudes require opportunities to become behavior; thus increasing the number or awareness of opportunities can increase the number of people who take advantage of them without relying on changes in attitude.

## PROVIDER FACTORS

Aside from demographic and psychographic features of the potential users of health services, plus their health-related behavior, attributes of providers are important determinants of health services use. As with people factors, provider factors fall into objective attributes (like demographics), subjective characteristics (psychographics), and behavior. The future state of all three categories of provider factors can have significant impact on health services use by the population they serve.

### Objective Characteristics

*Access*

A large number of characteristics of the health care delivery system affect the use of health services by specific populations. A major category among the objective characteristics includes all factors that affect actual access to care. This includes geographic access, convenience, and financial access. Beginning with comprehensive health planning legislation in 1966 (Public Law 89-749), great emphasis has been given to improving access to care for disadvantaged populations in isolated rural areas and core cities. With so much emphasis on cost containment, access is far back in second place, but significant progress has been made.

The government-stimulated increase in physician availability has forced young doctors to look to underserved areas as practice opportunities. Federal programs such as Rural Health Initiatives and National Health Service Corps have subsidized the development of programs serving underserved areas. Based on what we know about geographic access, we would expect that making care available closer to people would tend to increase their use of it, within limits. There still seem to be cultural factors that limit use even when access is improved, however.

Increasing access to care can also occur by making it available at more convenient hours or by reducing the waiting time for an appointment or the wait to be seen. The recent growth of walk-in immediate care centers (called *urgicenters, minor emergency centers,* or some similar names) demonstrates the attraction of a health service that can offer immediate access when people wish to be seen. Programs such as InstaCare® that guarantee 60-second response in emergency rooms reinforce the effect of convenience factors. Based on recent studies it appears that immediate care centers are not drastically reducing utilization of hospital emergency rooms. It is likely that they are competing with physician offices and actually increasing the use of care.

Financial access was the principal target of the Medicare and Medicaid legislation in 1965. It has long been recognized that ability to pay is a major psychological factor affecting an individual's likelihood of seeking care, especially when there are other options. It is also recognized that ability to pay is becoming an even more important concern for all providers who have to shift the costs from those who pay little or nothing to those who pay full charges. We seem about to create a dual-class system such as in Great Britain, with the poor being cared for by low-cost physicians who can get by on what governments will pay and the more affluent seeking care elsewhere.

Differential access affects the use of care in two significant ways. First, it affects the sheer volume of use and its characteristics. People with poorer access to care tend to use less of it, delay seeking care, and are sicker when they do. Hence Medicaid and indigent patients tend to require more intensive care, even controlling for diagnosis. Second, access factors influence where people seek care and which provider they prefer in terms of geographic convenience and financial access. From a forecasting perspective these factors must be recognized in estimating future use. From a management point of view they are all manipulable, hence can be used in marketing strategies.

*Insurance*

The type of insurance coverage that people have, as well as whether they have any, greatly influences care-seeking behavior. The deductible and co-insurance provisions reappearing in insurance coverage are specifically designed to reduce utilization, especially for marginal need situations. They tend to reduce or delay use whenever people feel that they have a choice. By eliminating coverage for specific untested or ineffective procedures, insurance companies can effectively dictate what sorts of treatments are used.

Insurance has a great deal to do with provider preference, as well. Provisions that cover services in the emergency room but not in the physician's office have been a boon to hospital emergency rooms. A reversing trend is apparent with insurance covering only those costs common to physician offices rather than the higher charges likely to prevail in hospitals. Coverage by an HMO plan, especially a closed panel group practice, virtually dictates where people seek physician services and often where they are hospitalized. Preferred provider organizations or exclusive provider organizations are being touted as the best way to control costs by directing insured populations to lowest cost providers.

**Psychographics**

Objective factors aside, the attitudes of providers, especially physicians, are another major factor influencing the use of care. The difference between what McClure calls aggressive and conservative practice has produced widely ranging patterns of hospital utilization. Wennberg and Gittelsohn have found wide differences in health care utilization, even among different counties in the same state. Family practitioners are widely held to be far less likely to hospitalize patients than are internists, for example, even controlling for patient condition. Physicians tend to use the technology in which they are trained, so the medical school residency training and age of physicians influence how they handle similar cases.

Provider psychographics and economics may work together to influence utilization. As the sheer number of physicians increases compared to the size of the population that they serve, each would expect to see fewer patients. In order to achieve a desired income level from a smaller practice, each physician must combine an increase in the number of services for each patient with an increase in charges per service. If price competition has any effect, it will increase the amount of procedures per patient that will be necessary. That such dynamics occur while we are trying to contain the costs of health care simply points out the inconsistency of government policy: increasing the number of providers while expecting costs to go down.

Hospital psychographics can also influence the pattern of preference in utilization. Hospitals that require or prefer more affluent or better-paying patients are moving to the suburbs, away from the poor-paying patients in core cities. In pursuit of more paying customers, hospitals are offering stress-reduction programs to executives and industrial health services to employees; both groups are virtually guaranteed to be able to pay for care received. Profit-motivated hospitals can refuse care to nonpaying patients or at least minimize the likelihood that such patients will seek them.

In general, provider psychographics, like those of consumers, are difficult to predict and subject to manipulation. Which hospitals accept, even reach out to, the poor may be predictable under current policies but subject to change if incentives are altered. Changes in physician training or sharing of risk may increase cost-consciousness to a significant degree. In any case how providers think and feel can have significant bearing on future utilization of health services.

**Environment**

Factors such as government reimbursement policy have been identified already as influencing utilization. Other environmental factors are important specifically because they influence consumers and providers in significant and predictable ways. Developments in malpractice, for example, have had great impact on provider behavior. Physicians have been forced to adopt more defensive medicine, performing tests or adjusting treatment specifically to protect themselves from possible malpractice suits. Hospitals have had to take a much more active role in ensuring that medical staff privileges are effectively managed and actively managing their own risks.

The state of the economy, especially employment levels and patterns, greatly determines the extent of insurance coverage in the population. Third-party reimbursement has a lot to do with the extent to which nursing homes, home health care, and other programs are available to be used. A vast array of environmental factors can and do influence the health of populations and thereby their probable use of health services. Cost-containment efforts and competitive pressures are likely to influence the relative use of different providers.

**IMPACT ON FORECASTING**

With such a vast array of factors known to be linked to the use of specific health services, the challenge of forecasting such use in a specific context is bound to be difficult. Added to this, however, is the fact that each individual factor is likely to be affected by or affect other factors. The dynamics of cause and effect in which these factors operate are likely to be complex and interactive rather than simple and unidirectional. Looking just at the categories of factors, for example, a graphic portrayal of their relationships would probably look like Figure 8-1.

**Examples of Interactions**

The following are examples of factor interactions:

- People demographics and provider behavior. Physicians keep people who live far away longer in the hospital because they know that they can't follow them up on an outpatient basis
- People behavior and people demographics. Fertility rates affect proportions of children; health-related behavior affects survival and proportions of aged
- Reimbursement and provider objective factors. Insurance reimbursement affects numbers of physicians by specialty through determining which are most economically rewarding

There are likely to be multiple examples of interactions among all variables affecting one or more types of health services use. The key is to focus on enough of the dynamics so as to anticipate important changes, while avoiding the need to consider so many factors and interactions that no sense can be made of them. If a single factor is so overpowering in effect or the only one whose future can be forecast, then future use may be predicated on, thereby predicted through, that one factor. If multiple

**Figure 8-1** Factor Relationships

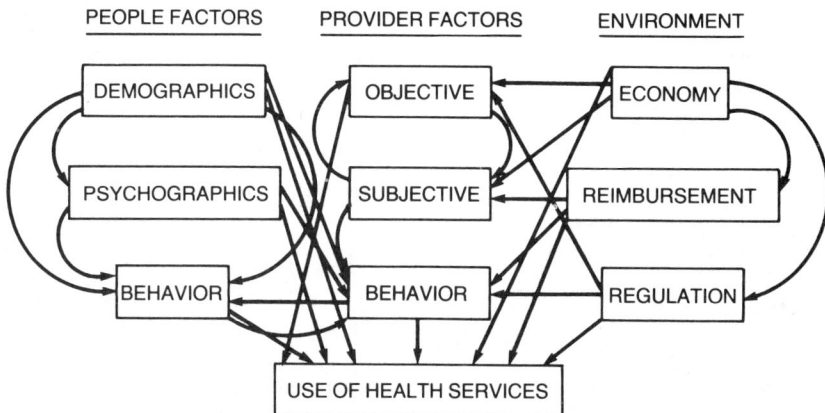

factors can and must be considered, some form of multivariate prediction technique would be called for.

## SUMMARY

In order to employ a prediction technique to forecast use of health services, it is essential to understand the causal dynamics affecting how a population thinks and behaves relative to such use. In addition, to make a decision based on a utilization forecast, it is necessary to understand the causal dynamics that determine how alternative decisions and potential utilization levels interact to affect the organization.

In general, causal factors related to utilization can be broken down into people factors, provider factors, and environmental realities. People factors include demographic characteristics of people who might use a specific service or provider and their ideas, psychographics. Demographic factors of importance include the numbers of people, their age mix, health status, ethnic identity, income and education levels, insurance coverage, gender, and residence. Psychographic factors include health knowledge, perceived health status, perceptions of health services and providers, and tendencies to behave in specific ways relative to health services utilization.

Provider or health system factors include objective and subjective attributes also. The access offered to people who might use a given service, involving geographic proximity, convenience, and financial access, is particularly important. How providers think and interact with patients is another important factor, affecting utilization during each contact plus the likelihood of future contacts. Significant environmental developments such as reimbursement changes, the state of the economy, government regulation, and legal developments can have significant impact on health service use. The full array of causal factors acts on each other as well as on health services utilization in some extremely complex ways.

---

**Annotated Bibliography**

**Aday, L., and Eichhorn, R.** *The Use of Health Services: Indices and Correlates.* Washington, D.C.: National Center for Health Services Research and Development, U.S. Department of Health and Human Services, 1981.
  Provides an excellent bibliography of works addressing the universe of factors affecting health services utilization.

**Anderson, J.G.** "Demographic Factors Affecting Health Services Utilization: A Causal Model." *Medical Care* 11, no. 2 (March–April 1973): 104.

**Joseph, H.** "Empirical Research on the Demand for Health Care." *Inquiry* 8, no. 1 (March 1971): 61.
  Discusses an array of factors found in research studies to affect the use of health services.

**Lambrinos, J., and Rubin, J.** "The Determinants of Average Daily Census in Public Mental Hospitals: A Simultaneous Model." *Medical Care* 19, no. 9 (September 1981): 895.

Examines factors affecting use of public mental hospitals, finding legal environment, availability of alternatives, prevalence of mental illness, and costs of services the best predictors.

**Levin, G., and Roberts, E.** *The Dynamics of Human Services Delivery.* Cambridge, Mass: Ballinger Publishing, 1976.

Describes the systems dynamics computer model as applied to forecasting the consequences of specific developments in the delivery of human services.

**Liu, B.** "Regional Hospital Needs Projection: An Input-Output Approach." *SocioEconomic Planning Sciences* 10, no. 1 (1976): 37.

Breaks down factors influencing use of inpatient hospital care into medical and technical factors and demographic attributes of populations.

**Newhouse, J.** "Forecasting Demand and the Planning of Health Services." In *Systems Aspects of Health Planning* edited by M. Thompson and N. Bailey. New York: American Elsevier, 1975, p. 87.

Cites health status and health insurance coverage of populations as better predictor than their socioeconomic characteristics.

**Rosenstock, I.** "Why People Use Health Services." *Milbank Memorial Fund Quarterly* 44, no. 3, part 2 (July 1966): 94.

A classic discussion of the impact of social and psychological factors on how people use health services.

Chapter 9

# Population-Based Prediction

The most powerful factor known in terms of predicting health services utilization is the size of the population. The sheer number of people served by an organization is the reality that best predicts its utilization; a change in the number of people served tends to have the greatest impact in terms of changes in utilization expected in the future. The second most important factor is the age mix of that population, both because changes in age mix can produce significant changes in utilization and because changes in age mix occur often. Gender mix is another important population factor but is less subject to significant change over time.

**USE RATE**

Because of the importance of population size and because population forecasts are likely to be both readily available and fairly reliable, the population use rate is easily the most common predictive technique used in forecasting health services use. The use rate is actually a mathematical ratio as well as a rate; i.e., it involves utilization per population as well as per unit of time. Thus, use rates may be expressed in terms of visits per person per year, patient days per thousand population per year, live births per thousand females age 15 to 44 per year, etc.

There are two basic ways to calculate use rates: the correct way and the easy way. Of the two the easy way is more common. It is exemplified by the old Hill-Burton use rate method for determining hospital bed needs. The total amount of utilization of health services in a defined area is first calculated. Then that utilization is divided by the population of that area. This is certainly the most direct way to calculate a use rate and the simplest, but it is likely to be incorrect.

A use rate by definition is the relationship between a characteristic behavior of a population and that population. The Hill-Burton approach describes the relationship between the experience of some provider organizations and a population. It assumes without evidence or analysis that (1) all people using an area's providers are residents of the area and (2) people who are residents use only those providers. The assumption is rarely true and may be grossly in error.

Such an approach to calculating a use rate may not produce erroneous results, provided one of two conditions holds. First, if the use of local providers by nonresidents and the use of other providers by local residents are both negligible, the error is minor. Second, if the use by nonresidents and out-of-area use by residents are close to equal, the error is also minor. The risk is that even where these conditions are true, erroneous forecasts can result.

If resident outflow and nonresident inflow are negligible and stay that way, forecasts based on use rates calculated in the Hill-Burton manner would not necessarily be erroneous. If either is substantial, error may be introduced in one or two ways. First, the pattern of inflow and outflow may change. More local residents may stay or leave; more nonresidents may use providers in their own area or more may come to local providers. Even if the tendency to use local versus out-of-area providers remains constant, however, different rates of growth in the size of local versus out-of-area populations would produce erroneous forecasts.

The population use rate is used as a ratio applied to a population forecast to produce a utilization forecast. Imagine a local population of 100,000 people and 300,000 visits to local physicians. Imagine also that of those 300,000 visits, 100,000 are used by nonresidents. The calculated use rate is 300,000 visits divided by 100,000 people, or 3.0 visits per person per year. Assuming that local residents obtain all their care locally (no outflow), their *actual* use rate would be only 2.0 visits per person per year.

Such a calculation would produce erroneous forecasts if the out-of-area population obtains its own sources of care and stops coming to local providers. If the local population is expected to increase to 200,000, the erroneous use rate would produce a forecast of $200,000 \times 3.0 = 600,000$ visits. If only local residents were to use local providers in the future, however, the actual utilization would be $200,000 \times 2.0 = 400,000$ visits. Moreover, if the pattern of inflow and outflow persists but the out-of-area population doesn't grow at all, expected utilization would be $200,000 \times 2.0 = 400,000 + 100,000$ out-of-area visits, or 500,000 visits altogether.

The only correct way to calculate population use rates and the only proper basis for using such rates in forecasting utilization require specifically incorporating inflow and outflow. Only through analyzing use of out-of-area providers by local residents and use of local providers by out-of-area residents can the true behavior of populations be identified. Once identified, the pattern of inflow and outflow can be examined and a specific decision made whether to forecast its persistence or change. Any difference in population change between local populations and those out of the area can then be specifically incorporated in forecasts.

Inflow information comes from the analysis of origins of patients using local providers. If 20 percent of all patients recorded using local hospitals reside in other areas, then inflow is 20 percent. This means that only 80 percent of local utilization is attributable to residents of the area.

Outflow is more difficult to determine. If patient origin data from all providers local residents use were available, it could be used to calculate outflow. Without such data a sample survey of local residents would offer a basis for estimating outflow. If 10 percent of all visits to physicians, admissions to hospitals, etc, are to physicians and hospitals outside the area, then outflow is 10 percent.

Inflow and outflow are percentages of different things, so they cannot simply be added or subtracted. Inflow is a proportion of all utilization *of local providers*. Outflow is a proportion of use *by local residents*. The denominators are different, so they can't be combined directly. If total utilization of local facilities were 100,000 patient days, for example, and 20 percent were used by nonresidents, then 20,000 of 100,000 days represents inflow. If 10 percent of all resident use of care went elsewhere, then 90 percent was used in local facilities. Because 80,000 days in local facilities represent use by local residents, then their total use of care was $80,000 \div .90 = 88,889$ patient days. Thus, the denominator for inflow is 100,000 patient days; that for outflow is 88,889 patient days. The use rate for the local population is 88,889 patient days divided by the number of people in that population, not 100,000 days so divided.

## AGE MIX

Given the importance of age as a factor affecting use of health services, the age mix of populations served is second only to their sheer numbers in forecasting. For different types of health services, different age mix effects would be expected, but age mix is likely to be significant for all services. Use of physician services is high for those 0 to 1 years, then diminishes with age through childhood. With adults, women use more services during their childbearing years. Older people use slightly more physician services with increasing age.

Nursing home services are used almost exclusively by those over 65. Use rates increase dramatically for those over 75 and over 85 and above. Hospital care is used far more by those over 65 than those under and more by adults than by children. The easiest way to express the effect of age is to employ age-specific use rates. The population should be divided into age segments within which use rates are homogeneous but across which they are significantly different.

For nonobstetric hospital care, for example, age cohorts used in age-specific use rates might be 0 to 14, 15 to 44, 45 to 64, and 65-plus. For obstetric care the female population should probably be divided into 5-year cohorts—15 to 19, 20 to 24, 25 to 29, 30 to 34, 35 to 39, 40 to 44—because fertility is sensitive to age differences within the 15 to 44 range. For nursing home care, populations might be divided into 0 to 64, 65 to 74, 75 to 84, 85 to 94, 95-plus, for example, to reflect the dramatically increasing likelihood of nursing home use with advanced old age.

If current age-specific use rates are known or can be readily calculated, they can be used simply to forecast utilization. Table 9-1 represents fairly typical age-specific admission rates and lengths of stay for the United States as a whole.

To employ these rates in forecasting hospital utilization, the number of people in each age cohort for some future year would be multiplied by the age-specific use rates. In considering whether to use the present use rates, it is wise to consider separately admission rates and length of stay. Only if both figure to persist unchanged or change in some coincidentally compensating fashion, will future age-specific use rates remain the same. Because age-specific population forecasts are likely to be available, this approach should be relatively easy to use.

There are times, however, when age-specific use rates are not available for the service population of the forecast. If age-specific population data for the present and forecasts for the future are available, however, there is a way to estimate the probable effect of changes in the age mix. Essentially it involves treating the local service population as if *changes* in the

**Table 9-1** Age-Specific Use Rate

| Age Group | Admission Rate | × | LOS | = | Use Rate |
|---|---|---|---|---|---|
| 0–14 | .070 | | 4.0 | | .280 |
| 15–44 | .150 | | 5.0 | | .750 |
| 45–64 | .200 | | 8.0 | | 1.600 |
| 65+ | .400 | | 10.0 | | 4.000 |

age mix have the same effect as in a reference population, even though its present use rate is different.

To illustrate, let us presume that the present service population contains 25,000 people aged 0 to 15, 40,000 people aged 15 to 44, 25,000 aged 45 to 64, and 10,000 aged 65-plus. Applying these figures to the age-specific use rates previously cited would yield the data in Table 9-2.

Thus, the expected local use rate would be 1.170 patient days per person per year, or 1,170 per thousand, as it is usually expressed. However, let us suppose the actual local use rate is only 800 patient days per thousand, or .800 per person. We can still presume that changes in the age mix of that population have the same *relative* effect as in the U.S. population used as a reference. To estimate the relative effect, we would apply the same age-specific use rates to the future local population and look at the results.

To illustrate, let us say that the future population will contain 20,000 people aged 0 to 14, 30,000 aged 15 to 44, 30,000 aged 45 to 64, and 20,000 aged 65 and over. Applying this new age mix to the same age-specific use rates would yield the data in Table 9-3.

Thus, if the U.S. population were going to see as much of a change in age mix as reflected in these data, we would expect a significant increase in use rate. Applying the same logic to the local population, even though it has a lower use rate than the United States, requires identifying the

**Table 9-2** Age-Specific Contribution

| Age Cohort | Population | Proportion | × | Age-Specific Use Rate | = | Age-Specific Contribution |
|---|---|---|---|---|---|---|
| 0–14 | 25,000 | .25 | | .280 | | .070 |
| 15–44 | 40,000 | .40 | | .750 | | .300 |
| 45–64 | 25,000 | .25 | | 1.600 | | .400 |
| 65 + | 10,000 | .10 | | 4.000 | | .400 |
| | 100,000 | 1.00 | | | | 1.170 |

**Table 9-3** Age-Specific Contribution

| Age Cohort | Population | Proportion | × | Age-Specific Use Rate | = | Age-Specific Contribution |
|---|---|---|---|---|---|---|
| 0–14 | 20,000 | .20 | | .280 | | .056 |
| 15–44 | 30,000 | .30 | | .750 | | .225 |
| 45–64 | 30,000 | .30 | | 1.600 | | .480 |
| 65 + | 20,000 | .20 | | 4.000 | | .800 |
| | 100,000 | 1.00 | | | | 1.561 |

*relative* impact of age mix changes on the U.S. age-specific use rates. The future use rate of 1,561 per thousand is 1,561 ÷ 1,170 = 1.334 times the present use rate. Assuming the same relative impact on the local population's use rate, we would expect it to be 1.334 × 800 = 1,067 patient days per thousand in the future. If no other factors were expected to alter use rates, that would be our forecast.

Once the use rate of the service population is known, we must still adjust for patient flows. If only 90 percent of local residents are expected to use local providers, we would multiply the population use forecast by 90 percent to get a forecast of how much use they will make of local facilities, the stay-home versus outflow proportion of their total utilization. To develop a forecast of inflow, a number of possibilities are available.

We might assume that inflow will remain a *constant proportion* relative to total local utilization. This is likely to be a simple but dangerous assumption in most cases. Unless the out-of-area population is changing in exactly the same way as the local population, both in size and age mix, and continues to travel elsewhere for care in exactly the same way as presently, we should not expect inflow to be a constant proportion.

If we know exactly where most of the nonresidents come from, we could analyze their population size and age mix in the same way as the local service population. After considering the likelihood of changes in their tendency to travel for care outside their area to ours, we could multiply their age-specific use rates times their population forecasts times their proportional outflow to us to determine the amount of utilization of our facilities expected. Adding this to the stay-home utilization of local residents would produce the forecast of total utilization in the area.

In most cases there is at least some inflow that we can't or simply won't bother to analyze. It might be patients from other counties, states, or even countries about whom we have insufficient data to make a systematic forecast. The conservative approach to such populations is to forecast the same *number* of patient days from them as in the most recent year, a constant amount rather than proportion. If we know that the population will increase by some proportion, we can always estimate that the amount of inflow will increase proportionately.

In general, service populations should be divided into two groups. One group, perhaps referred to as the primary service population, we will analyze systematically using age-specific population forecasts, use rates, and provider shares. The immediate local service population and any other nearby populations for which data are available and systematic analysis makes sense make up this group. When the same analysis is applied to all members of such populations, they are part of the primary service population.

For the remaining proportion of utilization, generally a small proportion (under 10 percent, preferably under 5 percent), we will not use the same systematic analysis. For reasons of lack of data or simply convenience, we will make some rough, preferably conservative, estimate regarding what they will contribute to the utilization of local providers. If their utilization is critical to making a decision, we should probably not treat them in this fashion but only if their utilization is incidental. This second group, not subject to careful analysis and forecasting, can be called the *secondary service population*. The difference between primary and secondary should be the difference in how forecasts of their utilization of local facilities are developed rather than any arbitrary definition.

Often a great deal of unnecessary attention is given to the identification of service areas or medical trade areas, however they are labeled. As long as the expected population of an area, its expected use of all providers, and its expected use of the specific providers about whom decisions are to be made are reasonably forecast, it makes little or no difference what populations are included or excluded. Populations who behave differently in their preference for specific providers should probably be examined separately, but this doesn't require labeling other populations as not part of the service population or even as part of the primary service population or trade area. In general, the finer the analysis in terms of separating populations that behave differently, the better the forecast is. This must be tempered, of course, with the realities of data availability and the added complexity of dealing with many separate populations.

The utilization of any specific provider is always a function of two rates. First is the rate at which populations served by that provider use the type of care offered by the provider. This is addressed by accurately measuring their present use and considering whether factors such as changing age mix will alter their future use. In the immediate and short run, significant changes are rare. The second critical rate is the tendency of the populations served to use one provider versus others: that provider's market share. This can change significantly in the short run and is subject to conscious influence by competing providers. Both rates must be addressed to get accurate forecasts.

## HMO POPULATIONS

A specific example of market preference that actually affects total utilization in an area is the HMO effect. It is generally found that populations enrolled in closed-panel group-practice HMOs use hospital care quite a bit less than other populations covered by conventional insurance. There is much debate regarding how such lower use rates come about, and even whether lower is better, but it seems clear that lower use rates are characteristic of HMO populations.

If HMO portions of a specific service population use care at a rate of 500 patient days per thousand and that the population as a whole uses 800 patient days per thousand, then changes in the portion of the population enrolled in the HMO would be expected to affect overall utilization. For illustration, let us assume that 10 percent of the service population is enrolled in the HMO. Because we know the HMO-specific use rate and the total use rate, we can easily figure the non-HMO use rate (Table 9-4).

We know from Table 9-4 that HMO populations contribute .050 to the overall use rate of .800. This means that non-HMO populations must contribute the remaining (.800 minus .050) equals .750. With 90 percent of the population contributing .750 to the overall use rate, their group-specific use rate must be .750 ÷ .90 = .833, or 833⅓ patient days per thousand.

If the 20 percent of the future population is expected to be enrolled in the HMO, the effect of this change would be estimated as in Table 9-5. Doubling the proportion of the local population enrolled in the HMO would thus be expected to cause a drop in the overall use rate of a little over 4 percent.

Care must be taken in making such group-specific adjustments. HMO populations generally include no aged members because enrollment is usually through employee groups. Thus part of the reason for a lower use rate by HMO groups would be that they are younger than the rest of the population. If a large number of people switch into HMO enrollment, the

**Table 9-4** Group-Specific Rate

| Group | Proportion | × | Group-Specific Use Rate | = | Group-Specific Contribution |
|-------|-----------|---|-------------------------|---|------------------------------|
| HMO | .10 | | .500 | | .050 |
| Non-HMO | .90 | | unknown | | unknown |
| Total | 1.00 | | | | .800 |

**Table 9-5** Estimated Future Group-Specific Rate

| Group | Proportion | × | Group-Specific Use Rate | = | Group-Specific Contribution |
|-------|-----------|---|-------------------------|---|------------------------------|
| HMO | .20 | | .500 | | .100 |
| Non-HMO | .80 | | .833 | | .667 |
| Total | 1.00 | | | | .767 |

age mix of the non-HMO population would tend to shift slightly toward the older, high-use cohorts. Thus the non-HMO population use rate might go up rather than remain constant.

If sufficient data were available, age-specific analysis of HMO and non-HMO enrolled populations would produce an estimate of this effect. The same sort of analysis described earlier to detect a shift over time would estimate the effect, even if the population as a whole expects no real change in age mix. Tables 9-6 and 9-7 might characterize such an analysis.

Changing HMO enrollment would produce an expectation that future non-HMO use rate would increase by a proportion of $1.380 \div 1.356 = 1.0177$. Applied to the present rate of .833, this would result in a non-HMO use rate of $1.0177 \times .833 = .848$. Applying this to the previous HMO analysis results in Table 9-8. This is in contrast to the unadjusted

**Table 9-6** Use Rate with Non-HMO Age Mix

| Age Group | Proportion | Age-Specific Use Rate | Age-Specific Contribution |
|-----------|------------|-----------------------|---------------------------|
| 0–14 | .20 | .280 | .056 |
| 15–44 | .40 | .750 | .300 |
| 45–64 | .25 | 1.600 | .400 |
| 65+ | .15 | 4.000 | .600 |
| | | | 1.356 |

**Table 9-7** Use Rate after Changed HMO Enrollment and Age Mix

| Age Group | Proportion | Age-Specific Use Rate | Age-Specific Contribution |
|-----------|------------|-----------------------|---------------------------|
| 0–14 | .20 | .280 | .056 |
| 15–44 | .40 | .750 | .300 |
| 45–64 | .24 | 1.600 | .384 |
| 65+ | .16 | 4.000 | .640 |
| | | | 1.380 |

**Table 9-8** Adjusted Overall Use Rate

| Group | Proportion | Group-Specific Use Rate | Group-Specific Contribution |
|-------|------------|-------------------------|-----------------------------|
| HMO | .20 | .500 | .100 |
| Non-HMO | .80 | .848 | .678 |
| Total | 1.00 | | .778 |

estimate that the future overall use rate would be .767. Clearly some analysis is called for to guard against missing an age-mix effect counter-balancing an HMO-enrollment effect.

## DIAGNOSIS SEGMENTS

A more complicated but potentially useful approach to segment-specific use-rate prediction involves categorizing the present and future population into diagnostic segments. This requires an extensive data base in which virtually all health services utilization by the population of interest has been recorded. With discharge abstracts or other medical records, all utilization is then characterized by the diagnostic-related-group (DRG) explaining each episode of use. Characteristics of utilization, e.g., length of stay per admission, are then linked to each DRG.

Current population data are then linked to utilization data to develop DRG-specific use rates for age-sex cohorts of the population. In effect this technique employs a cohort-specific use rate approach refined into DRG-specific use. Once present cohort–DRG-specific use rates have been determined, they are applied to population forecasts by cohort. The sum of all cohort-specific, DRG-specific utilization predictions then becomes the forecast for DRG-specific utilization by the target populations. The sum of all DRG-specific predictions is the forecast for total utilization by the population.

The DRG-specific approach, while substantially more complicated than a nondiagnostic-specific approach, is potentially far more useful. Knowing what shifts in diagnoses may occur greatly aids in predicting changes in patient acuity levels, staffing and equipment needs, and expected revenues and expenditures. It can be helpful in predicting the use of specific diag-nosis-linked services as well as overall utilization. It requires a substantial data base and extensive analysis but is likely to prove worth the effort. An example of this technique is described in Pekarna, D., et al., "Population and Diagnosis-Based Model Projects Bed Needs," *Hospital Progress,* January 1982, page 52.

Any identifiable segments of the population may provide a basis for developing a forecast of utilization based on segment-specific use rates. Three conditions are necessary, however, for this approach to prove successful. First, the population must be capable of being accurately described and forecast in terms of the segments. The entire population must be assigned to segments without double counting or missing people. Second, different segments must use health services differently, or it won't do any good to know how many people are in different segments. Third, the proportions of the population in each segment must be expected to change, or else there will be no expected impact on future use rates.

If these conditions are met, the segment-specific approach to predicting utilization usually provides good forecasts. The connections between numbers and attributes of populations and their use of health services is known to be strong and has been persistent. Changes in the connections have occurred but slowly and gradually in most cases, rather than dramatically.

As with all prediction techniques, using segment-specific use rates relies on the persistence of segment effects. Past relationships, no matter how strong and consistent, are not bound to persist, especially over the long run. Segment-specific use rate forecasts are likely to provide good estimates of utilization in the immediate and intermediate future. Some analysis and adjustment may be called for in the long run, however.

**THE COHORT EFFECT**

There is a significant risk in using age-specific use rates for long-term forecasting. This risk is based on what is called the *cohort effect,* i.e., the extent to which people born during the same period share experience or attitudes that make them significantly different from people born in other periods. To illustrate, consider the over-65 population in the year 1980. These people were born before 1916. It could well be that people born before 1916 share certain aspects of their diet, upbringing, or attitudes that make them substantially different from people born in 1916 and later. They may be more or less likely to use health services in specific circumstances or more or less likely to suffer specific diseases, for example.

If the people born before 1916 differ from those born later in ways that affect health service use, then the age cohort 65 and older may not use health care in 1990 exactly the way that the cohort used it in 1980. The over-65 cohort in 1990 may include more people born after 1915 than it will those born before. If there are substantial cohort differences, then age-specific use rates should not be expected to remain constant over a long period.

This is even more true where the members of a given age cohort change completely. In 1980, for example, the cohort of people aged 20 to 29 was born between 1951 and 1960. In 1990 the members of the 20 to 29 cohort would have been born between 1961 and 1970. Thus they are a completely distinct set of people. Chances are that people born in the 1960s are somewhat different from those born in the 1950s. If such differences affect their health status or attitudes toward health services, there may well be some impact on their use of health services.

## SUMMARY

Population—its size and characteristics—is such an important factor relative to use of health services that it should almost always be included as a causal factor in forecasting utilization, save for short-term situations. The population use rate is the most direct method for using the numbers of people served to predict utilization. The tendency for people in the defined service population to use outside sources of care and for outside residents to use local sources must be recognized in addition to use rates per se.

Among population factors most important to health services use, the age of the population stands out. Age-specific use rates or age-adjusted use rates that take into account changes in age mix represent the best ways of incorporating this vital factor. HMO membership is another factor that can be addressed in the same manner. A third factor, of particular importance in light of recent changes in reimbursement, is the diagnosis mix of the population served. Specific techniques for incorporating population factors in predicting utilization should be sought. Care should be taken to consider possible cohort effects as well as aging.

---

**Annotated Bibliography**

**Boffa, J., and Burck, M.** "Financial Projection in Prepaid Dental Care Plans." *Health Care Management Review* 2, no. 1 (Winter, 1977): 59.
Describes an actuarial approach to forecasting utilization of dental care based on populations of adults and children enrolled in a prepaid plan.

**Connecticut Hospital Association.** "Impact of an Aging Population on Utilization and Bed Needs of Connecticut Hospitals." *Connecticut Medicine* 42, no. 12 (December 1978): 775.
Describes enormous differences in age-specific use rates across populations and projects the impact of an aging population on use rates.

**Fisher, C.** "Differences by Age Groups in Health Care Spending." *Health Care Financing Review,* Spring 1980, p. 66.
Notes that the over-65 age group consumed nearly 30 percent of health dollars while comprising only 11 percent of the population, with roughly a third occurring in the last year of life.

**Fries, J.** "Aging, Natural Death, and the Compression of Morbidity," *New England Journal of Medicine* 17 (July 1980): 130.
Predicts that the extent of morbidity preceding death will diminish due to healthier life styles and medical advances.

**Griffith, J.** "Measuring Service Areas and Forecasting Demand." In *Cost Control in Hospitals,* edited by J. Griffith et al. Ann Arbor: Health Administration Press, 1976.
Discusses ways of identifying service populations and predicting their use of health care.

**Newhouse, J.** "Forecasting Demand and the Planning of Health Services." In *Systems Aspects of Health Planning,* edited by M. Thompson and N. Bailey. New York: American Elsevier, 1975, p. 87.

Describes attempt to use only demographic factors available through census data to predict use of health services; found them unsatisfactory.

**Pittinger, D.** "Population Forecasts for Health Planning: An Assessment of the State of the Art." *American Journal of Health Planning* 3, no. 1 (January 1978): 14.

Discusses techniques for forecasting the population and using age and sex cohorts to predict health services utilization.

**Reynolds, F., and Rentz, J.** "Cohort Analysis: An Aid to Strategic Planning." *Journal of Marketing* 45 (Summer 1980): 62.

Discusses the use of cohort analysis to differentiate the effect of becoming older from that of simply being in a different generation as it affects changes in behavior over time.

# Chapter 10

# Environment and System Prediction

Chapter 9 covered the use of attributes of the population to predict utilization by means of segment-specific use rates. This chapter discusses the use of environmental characteristics and health system factors to predict use of health services. The techniques used to relate environmental and system attributes to use of health services are different from those applied to population. They share, however, a critical similarity: both rely on changes in the predictive factors to produce changes in health services use.

## ENVIRONMENTAL FACTORS

The most important environmental factor relative to most health services utilization is the employment situation. This is true not merely because of the strong linkage between employment and insurance, or employment and health hazards, but because employment levels and patterns can change significantly in an intermediate and occasionally even an immediate time frame. Other environmental factors may have stronger objective links to use of specific health services but don't change rapidly or dramatically enough to be as important in forecasting.

One approach to recognizing the link between employment and use of health services is to treat such utilization as a function of the size of the labor force. Such an approach employs a factor strongly linked to both the size of the population and the level of employment. In prior studies the size of the labor force has been found strongly associated with use of inpatient hospital care, for example.

One of the difficulties with using labor force as a predictive variable is the difficulty of obtaining reliable estimates of what it will be in the future. If only wild guesses as to future employment are available, we might as well simply make a wild guess as to future utilization without bothering with the size of the labor force. The way to circumvent this problem is to use time-lagged rather than simultaneous relationships. This would mean expressing next year's utilization as a function of this year's (one-year lagging) or even last year's (two-year lagging) labor force.

The advantage in time lagging is that actual *measures* of the predictive variable can be used rather than forecasts. The disadvantage lies in the possibility that past time-lagged relationships may not have been consistent or the relationship may not persist. This is a problem shared with all predictive techniques, however, so time lagging may prove useful, at least for immediate range forecasting.

One key must be remembered in time lagging. The relationship to be used in forecasting should be exactly the same as that analyzed in the past to provide the quantitative basis for the prediction. Thus, if we are going to use the June estimate of this calendar year's labor force supplied by the state department of labor and industry to predict next year's utilization, we should use past June estimates and their relationship to their following year's utilization to calculate the predictive equation.

There may have been corrections made to the June estimates or other, more accurate estimates by another agency. That is no matter because the June estimate will be used to make a prediction. Use of corrected estimates would yield the wrong relationship to use in prediction and hence be likely to produce an erroneous forecast. Moreover the technique used by the source of the estimate to arrive at that estimate should have been consistent over past years, or the wrong relationship might result.

The relationship between labor force and utilization should be measured over a number of past years to determine its consistency. While one year is sufficient to calculate a relationship, it is risky if there is significant variability in this relationship from year to year. The calculation is simple, after all. If last year's June estimate of the labor force were 1.3 million and there are 2.5 million patient days of care used this year, then the ratio is $2.5 \div 1.3 = 1.92$. If past ratios have been 1.92, 1.86, 1.78, 1.98, 2.01, 1.74, 1.82, 1.88, 1.93, and 1.95, then the mean ratio is 1.887 and the standard deviation is .088.

If this year's June estimate of the labor force is 1.2 million, then the forecast of next year's utilization predicated on labor force would be $1,200,000 \times 1.887 = 2,264,400$ patient days. With a standard deviation of .088, we'd expect that about two-thirds of the time (68.26 percent, to be exact) next year's utilization should be within 1.887 plus or minus .088 times this year's labor force. This would amount to a range of $1.799 \times 1,200,000 = 2,158,800$ to $1.975 \times 1,200,000 = 2,370,000$. This range recognizes the variability of the predictive ratio in the past and thus an uncertainty over what it might be.

Any measurable environmental factor might be used in predicting health services utilization. It should be a quantifiable factor, of course, so that a mathematical ratio can be calculated between it and use of specific services. It should be logically related to use of services, so decision makers understand and have confidence in its predictive value. Most important, however, it should be expected to maintain its relationship with use of services into the future being forecast. For one or two years ahead at most, time lagging can make it possible to use known levels of an environmental factor to forecast levels of utilization. Beyond an immediate future, reliable forecasts of such factors must be available, which greatly limits options.

In addition to a simple ratio measurement, a linear regression may be used to describe the relationship between an environmental factor and health services utilization. The data in Table 10-1 might be the experience in a given area relative to emergency room visits and alcohol sales, for example.

The linear regression based on these 10 paired measurements is as follows:

ER visits = 1,074 + .329 × alcohol sales
$r^2$ = .939
standard error = 771

In contrast, a time series linear regression based on ER visits alone would yield the following values:

**Table 10-1**  Area ER Visits and Alcohol Sales

| Year | Number of ER Visits | Number of Gallons of Alcohol Sold |
|---|---|---|
| 1 | 40,000 | 120,000 |
| 2 | 42,000 | 125,000 |
| 3 | 45,000 | 130,000 |
| 4 | 42,000 | 128,000 |
| 5 | 45,000 | 132,000 |
| 6 | 48,000 | 140,000 |
| 7 | 46,000 | 135,000 |
| 8 | 46,000 | 138,000 |
| 9 | 50,000 | 150,000 |
| 10 | 48,000 | 145,000 |

$$r^2 = .758$$
$$\text{standard deviation} = 3,120$$
$$\text{standard error} = 1,535$$

i.e., more than twice the standard error of the regression predicated on alcohol sales.

Based on this analysis there has been a strong mathematical relationship between ER visit volumes and alcohol sales. It has been a consistent one ($r^2 = .939$) and would enable a fair level of precision in forecasting (standard deviation = 2,273, or less than 5 percent of the mean ER volume in the past). Deciding whether to employ this relationship in forecasting ER volumes should be based on a number of considerations.

1. Is this a true and direct relationship or a spurious one? It has been shown that a large proportion of trauma visits to ERs are linked to alcohol, but is this enough of a link?
2. Are forecasts of the predictive factor available? Can we obtain reliable forecasts of next year's alcohol sales?
3. Will the forecast be of sufficient precision for the decision that we're making? Is coming within plus or minus 5 percent to 10 percent close enough to plan staffing, budgets, revenues, or space?
4. Is the relationship likely to hold? Can we count on the persistence of this link or will other factors (e.g., growth in urgicenter competition, changes in health insurance) undermine the relationship?
5. Is this the best relationship available in terms of forecasting? Could it be that population is more closely linked to ER visits than are alcohol sales or that population forecasts are more reliable?

This last question is the most critical of all. Having what appears to be a good enough basis for forecasting shouldn't be the only criterion. Ideally the best basis should be used. In most cases a population-based approach should be evaluated first. Any other factor selected for consideration should have to compete with population, given its obvious logical link to health services utilization and generally superior potential to be forecast.

## HEALTH SYSTEM FACTORS

A number of health system factors are potentially well enough linked to use of services to serve as predictive variables. Principal among these are resource factors and access factors. All such factors enjoy the advantages of being logically linked to use of services and subject to conscious influence in attempts to affect as well as predict use. Selection of the best factor to use should be based on ease of measurement and confidence in persistence.

**Resource Factors**

The chief predictive factors in the resource category are the numbers, size, and types of providers available. The supply of physicians, both numbers and specialty mix, has a great deal to do with the amount and types of services used. The availability of specific alternative types of programs has great impact on the use of competing types of services. The supply of beds can certainly have impact on the use of inpatient care, though literal interpretation of Roemer's law is probably unjustified.

To some extent the availability of a particular resource determines its use. This is obvious when a given resource is absent, hence cannot be used. The Hill-Burton formula, for example, would always find the use rate to be zero in a county where no hospital existed. If left alone, such a use rate would guarantee that the county never had a hospital because its apparent use rate was zero. Although such an egregious error would be detected and corrected in most cases, similar but lessened effect results in areas simply short on resources. If the local hospital has only 50 beds, there are likely to be no more than $50 \times 365 = 18,250$ days of care used in that facility regardless of the size of the population. The share of total population's need for care served by the local facility would always be limited by the modest number of beds and probably related services available.

Making resources available may seem to "create" demand. There was certainly no demand for CT scans before 1973, when the scanner was tested at Mayo Clinic. The need, want, or desire for such a service must have at least been latent in the physician population, of course, or it would not have arisen when the scanners began to be available. Marketing has often been accused of manufacturing demand but can only take advantage of latent needs, wants, or desires in the population. Having competing resources available may make each more sensitive and responsive to consumer wishes, force lower prices, or otherwise tend to enable more latent demand to be realized. The idea that resources by themselves can bring about demand is an interesting one but contradicted by failures of hospital beds to remain full all the time, for example.

*Resource Example—Physician Supply*

The data in Table 10-2 might represent past measurements of the number of physicians on the medical staff and the number of inpatient days of care recorded at a hospital.

**Table 10-2** Medical Staff Size and Inpatient Days

| Year | Independent Variable: Medical Staff Size | Dependent Variable: Annual Patient Days |
|---|---|---|
| 1 | 121 | 36,000 |
| 2 | 130 | 40,000 |
| 3 | 128 | 40,000 |
| 4 | 137 | 42,000 |
| 5 | 149 | 44,000 |
| 6 | 156 | 48,000 |
| 7 | 150 | 45,000 |
| 8 | 161 | 49,000 |
| 9 | 168 | 51,000 |
| 10 | 175 | 55,000 |
| Mean | 147.5 | 45,000 |

A time series regression would have an $r^2$ value of .940 with a standard error of 1,419. It would predict that next year's patient days will be 55,200. In contrast a regression based on the medical staff size would have an $r^2$ value of .977 and a standard error of 878.5. It could predict next year's patient days only if a forecast were available of next year's medical staff size. If it were known that next year's medical staff will be only 150 due to the departure of a large medical group, a forecast of significantly declining utilization would make sense.

**Access Factors**

Any factor that tends to make it easier or more difficult to obtain health care when needed can be important in future health utilization. In general, access factors can be broken down into three main types:

1. geographic
2. operational
3. financial

Geographic access factors cover distance, topography, and transportation as they determine the ability to obtain care. Operational access factors cover the interactions between providers and recipients of care. Financial factors relate to the ability to pay for care.

Geographic access is affected by spatial distance and time of travel from where potential patients live and work to where needed care is available. In one noted study it was discovered that the likelihood of becoming a patient in a state mental hospital declined as the square of the distance from that institution. Travel distance is important, but so is access to transportation. For populations affluent enough to own cars or with ready access to public transportation, 10 or 20 miles may be a modest distance, although to others even a few miles may be too far.

Operational access covers all aspects of the interactions between patients and providers that influence how easy or difficult, convenient or inconvenient it is for such interactions to occur. The average length of time to get an appointment to see a specific provider is one such factor. The average waiting time before being seen is another, as is the time to get through a specific visit. Specific policies of a provider may make it easier or more difficult for some classes of patients. Regular patients are typically processed more quickly than new patients. Paying patients may be accommodated better than nonpaying. A quota or limit may be set for nonpaying patients, for example.

Financial access factors relate primarily to the prospective patients. The income levels of the population served and their insurance coverage are the major factors. Disposable income relative to service need can greatly influence whether people seek care and what form of such care (e.g., inpatient versus outpatient, institutional versus home care) they seek. Whether people have health insurance coverage and the specific coverage provisions of such insurance are critical factors relative to the type and amount of care people get. Deductibles and co-insurance, specific prohibitions or limitations can make dramatic differences in demand levels.

## HEALTH SYSTEM FACTORS IN FORECASTING

In contrast to environmental factors that can only be forecast, health system factors are subject to deliberate manipulation. Alterations in such factors can influence not only what types and amounts of health services will be used but also which provider of those services will enjoy what share of such use. With environmental factors the key is to anticipate changes in significant factors and estimate their impact on health services use. With health system factors such a passive approach may be unavoidable, depending on the scope and time frame involved. In many cases, however, the task is to estimate the impact on use of health services if specific changes occur, then to choose a change to pursue because of its expected impact.

Passive forecasts may be developed through linkages to health system factors in exactly the same way as with environmental factors. If the average physician generates 100 hospital admissions per year, for example, hospital admissions may be predicted by estimating the number of physicians available in the community and multiplying by 100. This simple ratio is identical mathematically to predictions developed through population use rates (Chapter 9).

Changes in the availability of one type of care may be used to predict utilization of another. It has been suggested, for example, that home care will substitute for nursing home care. If so, when no home care programs are available, nursing home use rates should be high. If programs become available, this should drive down nursing home use rates to some lower level but not below the point where such substitution does not apply. Similarly changes in the availability of nursing home care may increase or decrease the use of inpatient hospital care.

In such substitution cases there should be a mathematical function that sets the upper and lower limits on the use rates for one type of service and describes the impact of differing amounts of the substitute being available. For example, the function in Figure 10-1 might describe the relationship between the availability of nursing home beds and the use of inpatient hospital care.

Such a function indicates that shortages of nursing home beds can significantly affect hospital use rates but only below the level of 50 beds per thousand elderly. Having more than 50 beds per thousand available

**Figure 10-1** Relationship of Nursing Home Beds and Hospital Use

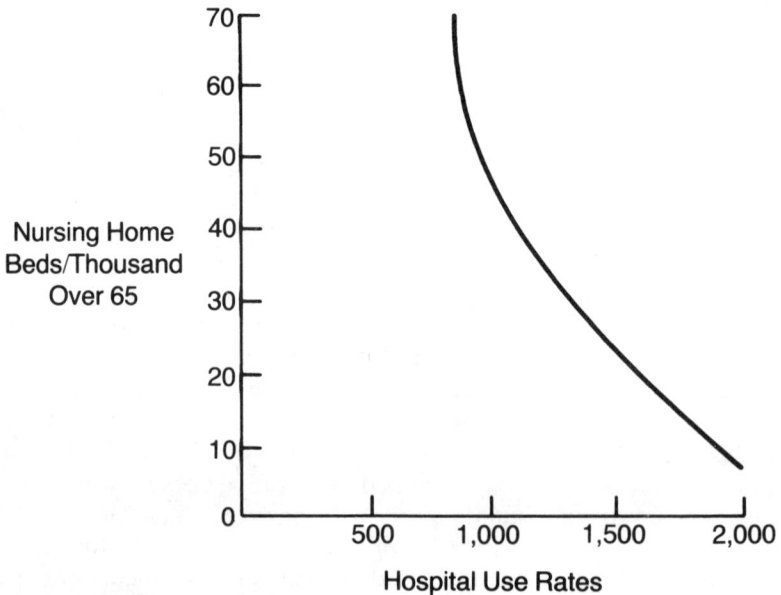

does not seem to result in lower hospital use rates. To the planner or policy analyst this would suggest the value of making enough nursing home beds available to prevent unnecessary use of inpatient hospital care. To the hospital, where inpatient use rates are high and nursing home availability low, it would be essential at least to estimate whether an increase in such availability is on the horizon.

Predicating utilization of health services on a single environmental or health system factor is simple mathematically but risky. Any such factor to which a mathematical value can be applied is potentially suitable for a predictive forecast. The future mathematical value foreseeable for such a factor must be either forecast or targeted for achievement. The relationships between values for any such factor and utilization of a specific service should be measured in a past time series or a present cross-sectional analysis to provide the measurement of the predictive relationship.

As with population factor prediction the consistency of past (or cross-sectional) relationships and their persistence into the future determine how effective any factor is as a forecasting base. Most useful factors have an obvious and intrinsic link with health services utilization, though the nature of that relationship may change while the link itself persists.

The availability of physicians has an obvious link to use of medical services, for example. On the other hand the predictive relationship might differ under different levels of availability. In the past, increases in the number of physicians have been generally followed by increases in the use of inpatient hospital care. In the future the opposite might be true. As physicians increase in numbers, their ability to derive the income desired from conventional practice comes into jeopardy. New physicians are responding by developing free-standing alternatives to hospitals for many types of services (e.g., ambulatory surgery, diagnostic imaging centers). Because patients must be ambulatory rather than inpatients in order to use these alternatives, physicians may increasingly find it both possible and beneficial to treat more people on an outpatient basis. Thus, an increasing supply of physicians may actually result in a decreasing use of inpatient care.

The biggest problem with using health system factors in forecasting is the difficulty in obtaining reliable estimates of their future value. As with population and environmental factors, it is possible to avoid this problem via time lagging, though this automatically dictates a shorter-term forecast at best. To forecast utilization two or more years ahead on the basis of health system changes is difficult in the more specific setting.

The best use of health system factors in forecasting is likely to be through simulation. If it is known that a given health system change would produce a desired utilization level, then efforts can be made to see to it that the change does occur. The initial forecast is a passive, hypothetical one, identifying what would happen to utilization if something happened to a specific factor. Once the simulation identifies which system factor to work with, an interventionist forecast is developed based on a commitment to achieving the necessary change in the health system factor selected (see Chapter 11).

## SUMMARY

A number of quantifiable factors may be used in predicting use of health services. These may be environmental factors, such as employment levels, or health system factors, such as the supply of providers, physical capacity of the system, or the relative access to care offered by the system. Such factors, to be useful, should have a logical and direct link to use of services, be measurable or forecastable with necessary accuracy, and have a persistent as well as consistent relationship to health services use.

In employing such factors in forecasting, either a passive or interventionist approach may be used, depending on whether the factor can be controlled or at least influenced by the forecaster in the time frame being forecast. In any event the factor selected as the basis for forecasting utilization should not only be strongly and reliably linked to health service use; it should be the strongest and most reliable factor available, and forecasts based on it should be the best estimates possible.

---

**Annotated Bibliography**

Ellwood, P., and Ellwein, L. "Physician Glut Will Force Hospitals to Look Outward." *Hospitals* 55, no. 2 (January 16, 1981): 85.
    Discusses impact of physician surplus.

Feldstein, P., and German, J. "Predicting Hospital Utilization: An Evaluation of Three Approaches." *Inquiry* 2, no. 1 (June 1965): 13.
    Discusses system factors such as insurance levels and hospital room charges and environmental factors such as urbanization on use of hospital inpatient care by state populations.

Kekki, P. "Analysis of Relationships Between the Availability of Resources and the Use of Health Services in Finland." *Medical Care* 18, no. 12 (December 1980): 1236.
    Offers insights from another country on relationships between availability of health resources and their use.

Long, M. "The Role of Consumer Location in the Demand for Inpatient Care." *Inquiry* 18, no. 3 (Fall 1981): 266.
    Discusses impact of geographic access to care on demand, controlling for demographic differences among urban, suburban, and rural populations; concludes that sociodemographic factors are far more important than place of residence.

Roemer, M. "Bed Supply and Utilization: A Natural Experiment." *Hospitals*, November 1, 1961, p. 36.

Discusses the Roemer effect, in which the creation of additional hospital capacity is followed by demand for more inpatient care.

**Weil, T.** "Do More Physicians Generate More Hospital Utilization?" *Hospitals,* December 1, 1981, p. 70.

Discusses growing surplus of physicians and cites three case studies regarding impact of changes in physician supply on use of health services.

Chapter 11

# Multifactor Prediction

With a complex phenomenon like utilization of health services, in light of the many factors that may influence such behavior over time, it makes sense to consider forecasting based on multiple factors rather than a single one. The more the factors recognized in predicting future utilization, the greater is the probability of incorporating significant changes. On the other hand the more factors there are, the more complicated the predicting process. When interactions among predictive factors are addressed, the process becomes geometrically more difficult as the number of factors increase arithmetically.

There are essentially three types of multifactor prediction processes, differing in how they deal with the predictive factors or independent variables. Econometric prediction treats factors in a series of mathematical expressions. Multiple linear regressions incorporate all factors in a single equation in which the influences of all factors are treated simultaneously. Systems dynamics incorporates not only the impact of predictive factors on health services utilization but the impact of utilization on the predictive factors and the interactions among the predictive factors themselves.

## ECONOMETRIC PREDICTION

As with any multifactor predictive process, the first step in econometric prediction is to identify the factors to be included. In recalling the variety of population, environmental, and health system factors that might be used to predict utilization (Chapter 8), it makes sense to select a workable number, no more than 5 to 10. Each factor must be capable of being expressed as a function of one of the other factors or as a direct predictor of health care utilization.

141

Essentially the econometric prediction process works backward from utilization of a specific health service, through factors that are strongly related to such utilization, until it reaches a factor that can be confidently and reliably forecast. If this tracing process is simple, the prediction process functions as if it involved only a single factor. In most cases, however, there are branches in the tracing process, and the effects of multiple factors are incorporated separately.

**Simple Econometric**

For example, imagine that utilization of ER services has been strongly linked to sales of alcoholic beverages. Unfortunately there are no readily available forecasts of beverage sales to use in predicting next year's utilization. However, imagine that alcohol beverage sales have been strongly linked to the number of males in the population aged 18 to 64. If a confident and reliable forecast of next year's population, male, aged 18 to 64, is available, it can be used to predict alcohol sales. This alcohol sales figure can then be used to predict ER utilization levels.

*Illustration*

ER visits have been shown predictable as a function of alcoholic beverage sales through the expression

$$\text{visits} = 5,098 + 2.858 \text{ (gallons of alcohol sold)}$$

Alcohol beverage sales have been shown predictable as a function of the number of males, aged 18 to 64, in the population through the expression

$$\text{gallons sold} = 10,124 + 2.163 \text{ (males 18 to 64)}$$

With a population forecast of 23,812 males, aged 18 to 64, in the local population, ER visits would be predicted as a serial function of the two factors:

$$\text{gallons sold} = 10,124 + 2.163(23,812) = 61,629$$
$$\text{ER visits} = 5,098 + 2.858(61,629) = 181,234$$

Because it is simple and linear, this relationship can be restated as a single expression:

ER visits = 5,098 + 2.858 [10,124 + 2.163(61,629)]

If the two relationships have held consistently in the past, it would be expected that there would be a strong relationship directly between the number of males 18 to 64 and the number of ER visits. Under such circumstances a direct expression of this relationship would easily be a more precise basis of forecasting than the two-factor serial function.

### Complex Econometric

In most cases econometric prediction is used because there is no direct, simple linkage from utilization of health services to a predictable factor. Instead there are two or more branches in the linkage, so that it is not possible to consider the utilization as a function of a single factor. Under such circumstances predictions of utilization are developed through applying as many mathematical expressions as needed.

For example, utilization of inpatient hospital care may be strongly linked to the size of the labor force, as suggested in Chapter 10. Rather than relying on a time-lagged relationship, a good forecast of next year's labor force might do a better job of predicting utilization. The size of the labor force might then be expressed as a function of interest rates and the relationship between wages and productivity. Interest rates might be predicted as a function of the size of the federal deficit. Wages could be a function of the previous year's cost of living index while productivity per worker could be a function of the average age of the worker, for example.

This complex set of relationships would be expressed in a series of mathematical functions. As purely hypothetical illustrations, these functions might be

- inpatient days of care = 1.462 × number of people in the work force
- number of people in the labor force = number of people employed in previous year ÷ (interest rate increase × wage increase ÷ productivity increase)
- interest rate = this year's average prime rate × .163 (rate of increase in federal deficit) and increase = next year's divided by this year's
- wage rate = 1.016 × this year's cost of living index ÷ last year's
- productivity increase = proportional change in the average age of workers from last year to this year × 2.164

If there are accurate measures and estimates plus reliable forecasts of the necessary predictive values in these functions, the expressions would be calculated in reverse order to produce the forecast of utilization. For example, the following series of calculations might apply:

productivity increase = $1.0063 \times 2.164 = 2.1776\%$
wage rate increase = $1.016 \times (267 \div 244) = 1.112$
interest rate = $.125 \times [1 + (.163)(.40)] = .133$
number of people in the labor force = $84,000 \div (\frac{.133}{.125} \times 1.112 \div$
1.021776) = $84,000 \div 1.158 = 72,539$
inpatient days of care = $1.462 \times 72,539 = 106,052$ patient days

If all the relationships were accurately determined and hold for one more year, this should be a good forecast. Each of the relationships is subject to past variation, of course, so there is probably a standard deviation associated with each. When applied in series, the standard deviations multiply. Thus the range of the ultimate projection could be quite large.

For example, the productivity increase expression might have a relative deviation range equal to plus or minus 5 percent. The wage rate expression might also be plus or minus 5 percent, as might the interest rate. If so, the labor force prediction could have a relative deviation range of roughly $\pm$ 15 percent ($1.05 \times 1.05 \times 1.05 = 1.1576$). If the labor force expression has a relative deviation of plus or minus 5 percent, then the prediction of inpatient utilization could have a relative deviation of plus or minus 21.6 percent. If the factors used in the predictive expressions are independent of each other, deviations should not be that large, but if they are linked, the final forecast may be too imprecise to be useful.

## MULTIPLE LINEAR REGRESSION

Rather than employing a series of mathematical expressions to deal with the impact of many factors, an attempt might be made to incorporate all important factors in a single expression. The multiple linear regression takes the same basic form as its simple counterpart, but with more than one independent variable:

$$y = a + b_1x_1 + b_2x_2 \ldots b_nx_n$$

This regression can take as many forms as the simple version. In fact each of the independent variables might be expressed in a different form, with one a simple multiplication, another based on logs, another based on squares, square roots, or division. Almost an infinite variety of forms is available, giving the multiple linear regression great flexibility but requiring a lot of testing to see which form works best on past data.

The first step in a multiple linear regression is to identify the predictive factors, the independent variables that are to be used in forecasting utilization. By recalling discussions of the dynamics affecting use of health services, selections might be made from any combination of population, environmental and health system factors. Feldstein and German, for example, forecast statewide hospital inpatient days as a function of inpatient versus outpatient charges, the proportion of the population over 65, and the extent of coverage by health insurance.

Whatever selection of factors is made, the next step is to obtain measurements or estimates of all factors for the necessary time periods. Normally this involves taking simultaneous measurements of all variables, independent as well as dependent. Because time lagging may be used for one or more of the independent variables, simultaneous measurement is not always appropriate. As with simple regressions, where measures of past periods in the place of interest are not available (time series), measures of present values in a number of different places (cross sections) may be used. The same risk applies to this expedient as applied to the simple regression, of course.

In order to have enough observations to produce a valid regression relative to past data, a larger number of observations is required than with a simple regression. Force fitting, i.e., guaranteeing a $r^2$ of 1.00, occurs in a linear regression when there are only two observations. For this reason it is wise to have no fewer than 5 and preferably 10 or more observations. The same phenomenon occurs in a multiple regression whenever the number of observations is equal to or less than the number of variables.

For a regression with three independent plus the dependent variable, force fitting occurs if there are no more than four observations, for example. In general there should be at least 5 more observations than variables, preferably at least 10 more. This helps assure that the regression at least accurately portrays past relationships among variables and accurately indicates the consistency of those relationships.

Another requirement in multiple regressions is that the independent variables should be, if possible, independent of each other. This is most important if an independent variable might be used to simulate the effect of deliberately altering its status in order to alter use of health services. If the size of the population and the number of physicians are to be used in predicting use of some service, for example, it should be recognized that the two tend to vary together. Typical regression software measures the covariance among independent variables as a check for this phenomenon.

Once the variables have been selected and the necessary sets of observations made, the next step is specifying the form of the regression. Because each independent variable may be expressed in a variety of forms such as logarithm, square, square root, and reciprocal, choices must be made for each variable as well as for the entire regression. With a computer a variety of forms may be tried to see which works best. This can take up quite a bit of computer time, however.

One way to select the form for each variable is to try each one in a simple regression first. If the simple, logarithmic, square, reciprocal, or exponential form works best for a given variable in a simple regression, that form is the logical choice for the multiple regression as well. Testing the best form for each independent variable requires little computer time, especially compared to testing all possible mixes of forms for the multiple regression.

Another choice with a multiple linear regression is the order in which the independent variables are introduced to analysis. The order does not make any difference to the overall value of the regression, but it can be important to identifying the most useful predictive factors. With a computer program and a relatively modest number of independent variables, all possible orders of variables can be tried in a stepwise fashion to see which have the greatest predictive value as they are added.

This stepwise regression approach produces measures for each variable as it is added to the analysis. At the point where adding one more variable produces little or no change to the $r^2$ value of the regression, it can be concluded that the best variables are already in. As with selecting forms of the regression, the identification of the best order for introducing variables in a stepwise manner can be assisted by examining the results of simple regressions, using each of the independent variables first.

A number of values indicate the potential of a multiple regression by describing its effectiveness relative to past data. The $r^2$ value for the regression, assuming that no force fitting has occurred, indicates the same improvement over knowing nothing about independent variables as true for a simple regression. The standard deviation of the regression indicates the degree of consistency in past relationships. The $F$-test value, derived from the $r^2$ value, indicates whether the results could have occurred purely by chance.

In addition to these familiar measures some unique to the multiple regression are equally important. One is the $t$ value for the coefficient applied to each independent variable. The $t$ value is a function of the coefficient and its standard deviation, as distinct from the standard deviation of the entire regression. The standard deviation of the regression indicates how much the results of the entire regression varied from actual values of the dependent variable through the multiple applications of the regression. The standard deviation of the coefficient indicates how much the value of that coefficient had to vary from application to application in order to fit the dependent variable.

If the value of the coefficient is close to or less than the value of the standard deviation, this indicates that the independent variable was not useful in predicting the dependent. For example, if the coefficient for some independent variable were 2.00 and its standard deviation 1.50, then the 95 percent confidence interval for that coefficient would extend 2.00 plus or minus 1.96(1.50), or roughly minus 1.00 to plus 5.00. Where this confidence interval extends into both plus and minus values, we cannot be sure even that its effect on the dependent variable is positive or negative.

The $t$ value is a measure of the usefulness of a single variable in the regression. For a given variable its individual value might be nil, but it still might contribute to the value of the regression as a whole. The contribution of each individual variable to the overall regression is expressed by the increase in the regression's $r^2$ value that it produces when added in a stepwise analysis. The $t$-test value indicates only how reliable a variable is individually as a predictor of changes in the dependent variable.

The strength of an independent variable, i.e., the amount of its impact on the dependent as opposed to the reliability of that impact is shown by the standardized beta value for each. The beta value indicates what percentage of change in the dependent variable is produced for each 1 percent change in the independent. The variables with the higher beta values tend to have the greater impact, based on past observations. The combination of beta values and $t$-test values indicate which variables are most valuable to the regression.

## SIMULATION

The importance of $t$-test and beta values is greatest when a multiple regression is intended to be used as a simulation. Whenever one or more of the independent variables are subject to deliberate manipulation, the regression has the potential for use as a simulation. Rather than merely forecasting values for the independent variables, hypothetical values for selected variables may be used to determine the impact on use of health services if a variable were to have a specific value. Alternative bed-to-population ratios might be tried to see if they would result in different inpatient versus outpatient use rates, for example.

A number of risks are involved in using regression results for simulation purposes, however. Regressions, like any correlation-based analysis, test only past associations. They cannot guarantee future associations, and they do not prove any cause-and-effect relationship. The number of beds may be linked to use of inpatient care because of more beds required by greater use of care rather than because of any Roemer effect, for example. If so, altering the bed supply may cause a change in inpatient use as far as the regression is concerned but have no such impact on reality.

To employ a given independent variable for simulation purposes, we must be sure that, first, we can manipulate that variable, and, second, if we do so, it causes or at least results in the expected change in the dependent variable. If the hypothesized values of the independent variable are outside the range of values used in the regression, we should be careful in predicting the consequences, for example. We should at least understand the dynamics that account for the regression-measured impact of any variable before we decide to use it as a device for altering utilization of health services.

The dynamics affecting use of health services might be more complicated than suggested in the regression. If so, while we deliberately alter a given variable in order to produce a desired level of utilization, some other variable, changing without our involvement, may entirely counter our efforts. Moreover, because of the probable interdependence among variables, deliberately altering one may not have the desired effect unless we also alter others.

## REGRESSIONS IN FORECASTING

The vast majority of multiple regressions mentioned in the literature have been used in prediction rather than forecasting. They have been applied to past data to explain why something changed rather than to anticipate how something would change. As a consequence the champions of regressions often neglect an important requirement for forecasting with a regression. Each of the independent variables must be susceptible to accurate measurement (in time lagging) or reliable forecasting in order to obtain the necessary values for predicting levels of the dependent variable.

It might well be that environmental values, such as labor force size, or system variables, such as hospital charges or physician supply, have strong and consistent association with use of health services. In order to employ these variables to predict use of health services, however, we need forecasts as to what *they* will be like. If the best we can do is to take a wild guess as to their future values, then we cannot expect the resulting prediction of health services utilization to be any good.

Because of this significant limitation, multiple regressions for forecasting purposes tend to be limited to short-term forecasts, with time lagging a common practice. Next year's physician visits might well be reliably predicted based on this year's physician supply, hospital ER charges, and insurance coverage, for example. Utilization during the year after next or beyond could easily be beyond the reach of regression forecasting, however. If population factors such as the size and age mix of the population are the only independent variables, a regression might well be used for longer-range forecasting. If all are population variables, of course, one of the simpler, population-based techniques described in Chapter 9 might do better and be easier to explain to the consumers of the forecast.

## SYSTEMS DYNAMICS

Both econometric and regression predictions assume a unidirectional flow of causality. That is, they assume that changes in the values for independent variables result in changes in the values of the dependent variable, use of health services. It must be recognized, of course, that the use of health services may cause some things to happen. In fact use of health services may have some impact on one or more of the independent variables. This feedback effect is simply not recognized in most forecasting methods.

One exception is a technique called *systems dynamics,* based on industrial dynamics developed by Dr. Forrester at Massachusetts Institute of Technology. This technique specifically addresses not only the interactions among independent variables but also the interactions between the dependent and all independent variables. As a consequence it is substantially more complicated but potentially far more useful than models based on a unidirectional flow of cause and effect.

For example, the use of specific health services such as family planning and contraception services, genetic counseling, fertility services, and abortions has obvious impact on each other and on the size and age mix of the population. The direct interactive effect has a significant time lag but is probably substantial when felt. Use of health services also affects disposable income levels because some of the costs come out of the user's pocket in most cases. Use of mental health services can affect attitudes toward health and perceived health status, which are known to have an effect on the use of health services.

Systems dynamics identifies the major factors involved in the complex cause-and-effect relationships affecting use of health services. It then describes the nature of those relationships in dynamic terms, indicating how a given change in one factor affects another. A positive link means that an increase in factor A tends to produce an increase in factor B (e.g., increase in average age of population causes an increase in use of inpatient care) and that a decrease in factor A causes a decrease in factor B. A negative link means that an increase in factor A causes a decrease in factor B (e.g., increase in number of urgicenters causes decrease in use of hospital emergency rooms) and a decrease in factor A causes an increase in factor B.

If there are sufficient data and understanding of the dynamics of complex relationships, systems dynamics calculates the mathematical relationships between all variables and through this describes the pattern of expected changes over time. This system has been used to demonstrate how law enforcement strategies tend to *increase* the use of illegal narcotics, for example, because of the complex set of feedback relationships involved in the narcotics system.

The overall process of systems dynamics cannot be covered here. For long-term forecasting on a large scale, however, it provides an important conceptual model of the complexities of causal relationships. It can be used to simulate the probable effect of major interventions such as changing reimbursement on use of health services and health care expenditures over time. It is potentially useful for policy analysis and likely to be more reliable than any forecasting technique that ignores complex feedback interactions.

## SUMMARY

In most cases a number of predictive factors are used to forecast use of any specific health service rather than a single one. Multiple factors may be used in a series of parallel, interrelated expressions via econometric methods. They might be used in a simultaneous, single equation through multiple regression. A third alternative is the use of a time-phased inter-active process called *systems dynamics*.

Econometrics first identifies factors associated with the use of a specific service, then develops expressions linking one factor to another. In its simple form, factors are linked in a linear sequence. A more complex approach links multiple factors through sets of parallel as well as sequential relationships. Each linkage is used to predict mathematically the future of one factor as the function of another, then finally the use of health services as the function of all.

Multiple linear regressions combine a number of predictive factors in a single equation. By combining them this technique predicts the consequences of changes in each factor on the use of health services in the context of changes in all other factors. The multiple linear regression is an excellent analytical tool, useful in identifying the dynamics and causal factors associated with health care utilization. Its limitations in forecasting arise from difficulties in obtaining precise, confident forecasts of the independent variables as the basis for predicting the future of the dependent.

Systems dynamics explicitly recognizes that relationships between identified causal factors and use of health services are complex and multidirectional rather than simple and unidirectional. It examines the relationships among all the predictive factors as well as that between them and use of health care. Although it is a far more complex approach to forecasting, it is also far more realistic.

---

**Annotated Bibliography**

**Beenhakker, H.** "Multiple Correlation—A Technique for Prediction of Future Hospital Bed Needs." *Operations Research* 13, no. 5 (September–October 1963): 824.
   Discusses the use of multiple regression to predict the demand for inpatient care in 17 specialty service categories.

**Campbell, R.** *Economics of Health and Public Policy.* Washington, D.C.: American Enterprise Institute for Public Policy Research, 1971, pp. 53–64.
   Discusses interactive effects of education and income on elasticity of demand for emergency, nonemergency, and preventive health services.

**Dove, H., and Richie, C.** "Predicting Hospital Admissions by State." *Inquiry* 9, no. 3 (December 1972): 51.
   Describes mix of population demographics, provider factors, and environmental factors used to predict hospital admissions by state.

**Feldstein, P., and German, J.** "Predicting Hospital Utilization: An Evaluation of Three Approaches." *Inquiry* 2, no. 1 (June 1965): 13.
   Examines three regression techniques used to forecast statewide hospital use; found the simpler alternatives better.

**Gutkin, C.** *Use of a Multiple Regression Model to Predict Hospital Outpatient Visits.* New York: Columbia University Center for Community Health Systems, 1973.
   Describes multiple regression model used to predict outpatient visits to a rural hospital in New York state, mixing population and provider factors.

**Moore, W., and Bock, H.** "Estimating the Demand for Medical Care." *Inquiry* 9, no. 4 (December 1972): 64.
   Describes the development of a computer-based simulation model using multiple linear regression to predict demand for a variety of health services in Texas.

**Rosenthal, G.** *The Demand for General Hospital Facilities.* Chicago: American Hospital Association, 1964.
   Examines a variety of ways to predict utilization of hospital care and concludes that a multiple linear regression works best.

**Siler, K.** "Predicting Demand for Publicly Dispatched Ambulances in a Metropolitan Area." *Health Services Research,* Fall 1975, p. 254.

Describes multiple linear regression used to predict demand for emergency transportation in Los Angeles.

**Stearns, N. et al.** "Systems Intervention: New Help for Hospitals." *Health Care Management Review* 1, no. 4 (Fall 1976): 9.

Describes systems dynamics concepts and techniques together with possible applications to specific hospital problems.

**Wan, T., and Yates, A.** "Prediction of Dental Services Utilization: A Multivariate Approach." *Inquiry* 12, no. 2 (June 1975): 143.

Describes a regression based on residence, religion, income, race, social class, and supply of dentists to predict use of dental services in New York and Pennsylvania through the use of the automatic interaction detector (AID) technique.

# Part IV

# Prospection Techniques

In contrast to projection and prediction techniques, which are imbedded in the past, prospection techniques look only forward. They "foresee" the future rather than calculate it as a function of past realities. It is entirely possible and often effective to estimate health services use without any data whatsoever about past use. Because there are many situations in which past data are unavailable or unreliable, prospection techniques are necessary in any comprehensive armamentarium of forecasting approaches.

An additional approach to prospection involves combining different techniques or even different forecasts in order to produce a judgment-based estimate of future utilization. Ideally, combining approaches should exploit the strengths and overcome the limitations of individual techniques. No single technique is likely to be so acceptable, precise, and accurate in practice as to warrant discarding all others.

Techniques may be combined in a variety of ways. One technique may be used to develop forecasts of factors used in another. For example, Delphi (Chapter 12) could be used to forecast a value to be used in a use rate approach (Chapter 9). By the same token future use rates could be projected via linear regression (Chapter 4) and applied to population. Delphi could be used to forecast individual factor impacts in a change factor approach (Chapter 13).

Another combining approach involves breaking down total utilization into its components, forecasting each component separately, then summing to yield an overall forecast. Hospital patient days could be broken down by service unit and into admissions and length of stay, for example. Clinic visits could be broken down into a forecast of the numbers of people using the clinic times their average number of visits per year. If separable components of utilization are subject to separate dynamics, then addressing and forecasting them separately tends to produce superior forecasts.

Finally forecasts derived from different techniques can be combined if no single technique seems overwhelmingly superior. Arithmetic means or medians may be used to develop an average forecast. Weights may be given to forecasts considered more probable or all may be treated equally. A PERT (program evaluation and review technique) convention adds the highest forecast, the lowest, plus four times the most probable forecast, then divides the sum by six to produce a combined forecast.

Selecting a way of combining forecasts is clearly a subjective process, even if all the techniques used in the combination are objective. This simply confirms the inherent subjectivity of all forecasting. Given the wide variety of techniques available, none of which have proven consistently superior to all others in all situations, there is always a requirement for subjective judgment. Such judgment may be used in selecting the techniques to be used, in choosing the data to be employed, in modifying results, in producing the forecast, or in combining multiple forecasts. This subjectivity should be recognized as an essential and valid aspect of forecasting rather than something to be reduced as much as possible through quantitative machinations.

Prospection includes the possibility of using projection and prediction techniques and results rather than representing an entirely separate approach to forecasting. In essence all forecasting is prospection, where any thought is given to future developments as a basis for selecting or adjusting a specific technique. Techniques may fall into one category or another, but the process actually used to forecast health care utilization should always be a prospection process. Because subjective judgment is always involved in forecasting, if only in choosing what data to incorporate and what technique to employ, all forecasting is subjective. Reliance on fallible human judgment is inherent in forecasting, regardless of the technique selected.

Chapter 12 discusses naive prospection, forecasting techniques that require no explicit understanding of the dynamics affecting health services use. They do not prohibit casual insights; they merely do not depend on explicit insights. The familiar Delphi technique is easily the best known of naive prospection methods, but others are available. The numerous modifications available for Delphi offer a variety of options in themselves. In addition analog forecasts and user surveys can be used. Both are independent of understanding why people use health services, though both require information about actual use to forecast the future.

Chapter 13 describes a systematic thinking process used to foresee health service use based on explicitly identified causal factors. Change factors enable forecasters to estimate utilization based on identified developments expected to occur without relying on patterns of past developments. By careful selection of factors, informed estimates of their change, and educated guesses about the impact of such changes, forecasters can develop reasonable and explainable forecasts of use of specific health services.

# Chapter 12

# Naive Prospection

Prospection techniques require only the ability to anticipate developments and their probable impact on use of health services. They rely only
on past experience, knowledge, and intuition rather than systematic analysis of past data. Four principal categories of naive prospection techniques
are covered in this chapter. The Delphi technique is a formal group process
for developing consensus estimates of the future. Analog forecasting rests
on the identification of specific experience in another time or place that
can be used to estimate future health services consequences. Scenario
forecasting develops alternative descriptions of possible situations as a
basis for foreseeing health services utilization, depending on which situation actually occurs. User surveys ask potential users of services to
forecast their own utilization.

## THE DELPHI TECHNIQUE

The Delphi technique, as perfected by researchers at the Rand Corporation, is a way of quantifying subjective estimates of the future. It begins
by selecting a group of people who are experts or at least reasonably
knowledgeable in areas thought important to future utilization of health
services. Each member of the group is asked to estimate the future value
for some specific utilization measure such as the population use rate of
inpatient care for the United States five years from now. Each member of
the Delphi panel arrives at an independent estimate of this measure without
consulting with other members or even knowing who they are.

Participants should represent whatever geographic area is the target for
prospection. If national use rates for hospital care are to be forecast,
participants should come from all parts of the country. If statewide rates
are to be estimated, participants should be drawn from throughout the

state but no further. For local use rates, local participants are preferred for both technical and political reasons. Participants must be familiar enough with the situation to forecast its development. Moreover participants from beyond the boundaries of the situation may be dismissed as irrelevant and immaterial by consumers of the forecast unless the participants are widely acknowledged experts.

These future estimates may in fact be derived in whatever manner each member sees fit. One may use a computer; another may apply a paper and pencil or hand calculator; still another may gaze into space and wait for a vision. Each member is free to develop an estimate in whatever manner seems appropriate. The Delphi forecast is simply a consensus estimate developed through the knowledge and insights of all participants.

Once each member of the Delphi panel has contributed a forecast based on prospection, mathematical analysis is applied to the results. The mean of all forecasts is calculated together with the standard deviation. These statistical measures of the average opinion and variability among opinions are then transmitted to all participants. Each member is asked to reconsider the original forecast. Those whose forecasts differed significantly from the mean are asked to explain why their opinions are so different.

The reconsidered forecasts, together with the justifications of outliers, are assembled for further analysis. New means and standard deviations are calculated and examined. If there has been significant movement, i.e., changes in opinion, the process might be repeated. If not, and it seems likely each participant will hold on to the original forecast, the mean of their estimates can be used instead of waiting for consensus.

**Modification of Delphi**

In practice the classic Delphi process is typically modified in one or more ways. In the true Delphi, for example, participants never meet or even learn the identities of other participants. This is intended to prevent dominance of a few by force of personality or reputation. It is also economical if participants live a great distance from each other. In addition it prevents conflicts that might occur during face-to-face meetings.

In many situations, however, it is useful, either technically or politically, to have participants meet. In order to preserve the spirit of Delphi, one requirement is essential. The first forecast from each participant should be developed, recorded, and submitted before any face-to-face discussion. This ensures that each participant has an equal voice in at least the first group estimate. It also reduces the likelihood of dominance by a few because each person is on record with a position to explain, if not defend.

Once the initial forecasts are in, any number of modifications can be made in the basic Delphi process. All participants may meet in a group to brainstorm their differences and pursue consensus. If the number of participants is large, i.e., more than 8 to 10, they may be more effective in smaller groups. Consensus reports from each subgroup may then be presented to the entire group of participants for further consideration. As in the basic Delphi, if consensus isn't reached, the mathematical average or median of the group's individual forecasts may be used.

Another possibility is to use remote communication for the first round, then have participants meet to discuss each other's forecasts. Each participant could be invited to bring along specific data or analyses that bolster each position. Such an approach would take advantage of the beneficial aspect of group conflict: it increases at least the quantity of information brought into discussion. The use of outside "evidence" may make it more difficult to reach consensus, but it would expose participants to more than merely other people's opinions.

If forecasting utilization requires estimating more than one specific value, Delphi may be used to develop consensus forecasts of each component. Hospital admissions could be forecast by one Delphi group, then length of stay could be forecast by another, after reviewing the admissions forecast. The same group might be used to forecast each but at separate times or even at the same time. If different types of people are likely to be informed better about pediatric utilization in contrast to obstetrics, for example, separate Delphi groups would be appropriate.

Multiple Delphi groups might be used in particularly sensitive situations. If a number of different groups arrive at roughly the same forecast independently, greater confidence might be placed in the result. However, if groups differ widely, substantial concern would be legitimate. The reasons cited by one group may be more persuasive than those of another, of course, making it possible to have greater confidence in one group's consensus than another's.

Based on experience with Delphi in forecasting, a few things should be kept in mind in designing and employing this process. The first relates to the selection of participants. It appears to make little difference to the ultimate accuracy or validity of forecasts if the participants are recognized experts in their fields or simply well-informed journeymen. The results from such groups tend to be about the same. There are times when it makes political sense to employ experts so as to lend an aura of objective expertise to a forecast. At other times using local talent makes better political sense and equal technical sense.

Another aspect of selecting participants relates to their homogeneity versus heterogeneity. In general the more alike the participants are, the less trouble they have in reaching consensus. On the other hand the more alike they are, the greater the chance their forecast may be significantly off. Physicians forecasting use of their services may share the same optimistic bias and be less sensitive to environmental factors, for example. Selecting participants from a variety of backgrounds increases the likelihood of conflict but tends to result in more accurate forecasts.

A third finding based on experience with Delphi is that in most cases there is relatively little difference between the median of initial forecasts and the final consensus forecast of the group. It appears that people alter their opinions somewhat in response to group norms, but this tends to be simply gravitation toward the mean. As a result the mean or median of the group's estimates usually does not change much. Unless the initial estimates have a median near a sensitivity level (Chapter 17), it often suffices to use the first round of Delphi forecasts rather than to pursue consensus.

If a modified Delphi, involving group interaction, is to be used, a second round of estimates is essential as the focus for group discussion, however. In managing group interaction, efforts should be made to promote participation by everyone. Each participant, especially those with estimates significantly different from the rest, should be given ample opportunity to explain each forecast. It is always possible that one or a few were sensitive to an aspect of the dynamics affecting use of health services that others ignored.

An essential data base for Delphi forecasting is often forgotten in practice but is absolutely essential. That is an accurate measurement of the most recent status of whatever utilization is to be forecast. All participants should start from exactly the same base, even if they bring to the process a variety of attitudes and insights.

### Applications of Delphi

The Delphi process is almost always used for longer- rather than shorter-range forecasts. It is likely to be useful in forecasting use of health services in periods 10 or 20 years from the present. It may in fact be the only approach possible for far-future forecasting, e.g., into the twenty-first century. It is especially useful when forecasts must be developed for situations in which there are no past data, such as for a new health service or new technology, even though a relatively short-term forecast may be involved.

Delphi is also useful in at least two other aspects of the forecasting process. First, Delphi may be used to develop an estimate of the present situation, should it be unsusceptible to timely and accurate measurement.

Psychographic realities, the attitudes of people, may be too difficult to measure or require more time and resources to measure than are readily available. If it is necessary to estimate present attitudes toward use of health services in order to forecast use, the Delphi process may be used. It is especially wise to use participants from a variety of backgrounds whenever Delphi is used to estimate present reality.

In addition to estimating the present, Delphi may be used to identify the sensitivity level or range for a forecast. Before any forecasting process is used, the group may be asked to specify what future utilization should be in some period. As discussed in more detail in Chapter 17, this sensitivity level can then be used to examine forecasts of utilization or serve as the basis for developing such forecasts.

## ANALOGS

Analogs are conscious models based on experience in another place or time. They are based on past realities, so in a sense are not fully prospective techniques. They are essentially and more obviously subjective approaches to forecasting, however, and so fit better into the prospective category than any other. They depend on the correct identification of the appropriate analog and the proper estimation of how the analog will apply to the future.

The basic logic of an analog is that some experience in this place or experience in some similar place is *just like* what will happen here. The pattern of sales of color television sets in this country was forecast based on experience with black-and-white sets, for example. The implementation of nuclear magnetic resonance (NMR) in the United States is likely to follow a similar pattern as sales of CT scanners in the 1970s.

To forecast use of health services by means of an analog, all that is necessary is that a proper experience be chosen. If the use of a new walk-in urgicenter in the north end of town is to be forecast, it would help to have the experience of one opened a year earlier in the south end of town, for example. If such an analog is not available, the experience of a similar program in a similar community could be used. If a good analog is not available from a similar situation, the average of similar programs in a number of communities could be employed.

In a way the innovation adoption curve, described in Chapter 7, is an analog because it is based on actual experience with similar situations. Rather than relying on finding a mathematical or statistical formula to describe the pattern of utilization experience in a similar program, an analog may simply overlay that experience on the situation to be forecast.

The key to effective use of analogs is the ability to identify a truly analogous situation. The experience of CT scanners may not be a perfect analog for the NMR because they are useful in somewhat different types of cases. Moreover the NMR is not quite as revolutionary a technology as the CT scanner and may be adopted more quickly. Conversely the NMR is more expensive than the CT scanner and may be adopted more slowly. Moreover, Certificate of Need refutation and payment system changes will probably have some impact. To be a perfect analog, the dynamics affecting the pattern of use must be almost identical in the past and future cases.

Experience of utilization in the north-end urgicenter may not replicate that of the south end, even if opened a year apart, for a variety of reasons. The population demographics or psychographics may be different. There may be a greater or lesser availability of competing providers in one place versus another. In fact the opening of the south-end center may have caused changes. People in the north end may have heard about it and become favorably predisposed toward its use. Conversely physicians in the north end may have heard about the success of the south-end center and have extended their office hours so as to make themselves more competitive in anticipation of such a center opening nearby.

With the analog approach it is essential, as in all forecasting, to understand the dynamics affecting use before forecasting utilization. The match needed for an effective analog forecast is one in the dynamics affecting utilization more than in the type of service to be used. If the dynamics in a different time or place were enough like the situation to be forecast and if they operate in the same way in the future, the analog will serve well in forecasting. If not, it becomes an uneducated guess that may be afforded more credibility than it deserves simply because it is based on objective past reality.

## SCENARIO FORECASTS

Scenario forecasting is based on identifying one or more critical factors, relative to use of health services, where the future is expected to take one of two or more substantially different forms. Based on each set of alternative future states of such factors, separate forecasts are developed. These forecasts are then compared to see how different they are. If they are sufficiently different to suggest that a different present decision should be made, a choice must be made as to which scenario is more likely and what risk the organization is willing to take. If it is possible to undertake effort in order to improve the chances of a desired scenario, a choice might be made in that direction also.

The first step in scenario forecasting is to select the factors whose future states are critical relative to the use of health services to be forecast. The number of factors must be kept to a manageable number, preferably less than 6, or it becomes extremely complicated to consider all possible scenarios. If there are 10 factors, for example, each of which can have three distinct future states, and if the factors are independent of each other, there would be $3^{10} = 58,049$ possible scenarios. Even with 5 factors, each of which could take two distinct futures, there would be $2^5 = 32$ possible scenarios.

In practice, critical factors are likely to be few and are also likely to be interdependent. In most cases there are likely to be fewer than six alternative scenarios sufficiently different from each other and sufficiently likely to be worth considering. To keep the number manageable, the number of factors and futures needs to be kept low.

To illustrate, in considering the future use of outpatient surgery, there might be identified three critical factors:

1. the ratio of surgeons to population
2. the type of coverage for outpatient surgery
3. the extent of pressure by government and industry to keep utilization to a minimum

The future state of these factors might be arrayed in the following choices:

1. surgeon ratio
   a) same as present
   b) 10 percent higher
   c) 20 percent higher
2. availability of coverage
   a) full coverage
   b) deductibles and co-insurance required
3. pressure
   a) modest
   b) extreme

Treating these factors and futures as independent, there would be $2^2 \times 3 = 12$ different mixes of the alternatives, or 12 scenarios. Some of these might be eliminated as unlikely groupings based on the following logic:

- Pressures to contain costs will be intense because there are too many physicians and would result in absence of full coverage, so (1b) and (1c) do not fit with (2a) and (3a).
- Deductibles and co-insurance are specific examples of pressure, so fit with (3b) but not (3a).

With these exclusions, the number of scenarios is reduced to four:

1. Stable surgeon supply
   a) full coverage
   b) modest pressure
2. Stable surgeon supply
   a) deductibles and co-insurance
   b) extreme pressure
3. 10 percent increase
   a) deductibles and co-insurance
   b) extreme pressure
4. 20 percent increase
   a) deductibles and co-insurance
   b) extreme pressure

Forecasts would be developed in light of the anticipated impact of the four combinations. In general it would be expected that increases in surgeons would be accompanied by corresponding increases in surgery. Assuming that this increases the overall surgery to population ratio, one would expect the additional surgeries to be of a less serious nature. If 25 percent of all surgeries are being done on an outpatient basis at present but 50 percent of the additional surgeries will be outpatient, then outpatient surgery increases more than the 10 percent or 20 percent increase in surgeons.

This can be analyzed with the following mathematics:

- Current surgery is split 75-25 so rate is equivalent of 75 inpatient and 25 outpatient
- A 10 percent increase in the rate would mean an overall rate 110 percent of the present. With half the 10 percent increase outpatient and half inpatient, the new split is 80 inpatient and 30 outpatient.
- A 20 percent increase would mean an overall rate 120 percent of the present, which would be split 85–35.

Therefore, with a 10 percent increase in surgeons, we would expect the outpatient rate to increase by a ratio of 30 to 25, or 20 percent. With a 20 percent increase in surgery we would expect the rate to increase by a ratio of 35 to 25, or 40 percent. Both other factors tend to reduce surgery rates, however, so would tend to counter this increase. On the other hand, if deductible and co-insurance apply equally to inpatient and outpatient surgery, there might be a tendency to shift toward more outpatient, where the out-of-pocket cost to the patient would be less.

A general group discussion might be used to estimate the combined effect of the four scenarios. Given the counterpressures involved, the outpatient surgery rates might be relatively similar under all four. On the other hand increases in surgeons and insurance charges might work together to increase outpatient surgery as an alternative to inpatient. Whatever is judged the most reasonable impact for each scenario would be used. A Delphi process could be used here, for example, to select the most probable outcome for each.

If the volumes of outpatient surgery expected to accompany the different scenarios are significantly different *and* if they would lead to different decisions in the present, then some further consideration is needed. If all are similar enough to point to the same decision, however, the process has served its purpose, and the decision can be made.

When further consideration is required, the task becomes estimating the probabilities of the four scenarios. Recognizing that the sum of the four probabilities must equal 1.00, each might be assigned a probability of .25 for starters. Discussion can then focus on which have greater or less than chance probabilities and by how much. Here again a Delphi process may be used to arrive at consensus probability estimates. Once the probability of each scenario is estimated, decisions can be made accordingly.

## USER SURVEY

A common marketing approach to forecasting use of health services is to ask those who will be users, and determine use from what they themselves see in their futures. Instead of asking physicians how many physician visits they foresee for an entire population via Delphi, for example, we could ask individual physicians how many of their own patients they intend or expect to refer to some clinic. Instead of asking some consumers on a panel to estimate consumer demand for an urgicenter, we could ask individual consumers whether they intend to use that program.

This approach is pure prospection in that it asks people to foresee their own behavior. It is a more systematic and scientific approach to prospection than other techniques in that it is usually carried out through a systematic sample survey of potential users. The results of this survey can then be used to infer what the entire population will do. Such surveys are subject to all the strengths and limitations of statistical analysis.

In contrast to surveys intended to sample a population about what is presently true, however, intention surveys are subject to an additional limitation. In foreseeing their own behavior, respondents to the survey may not prove good forecasters of even their own behavior. If only 50 percent of the people who *say* that they will use a specific service actually do so or if 50 percent of those who indicate that they *do not* intend to use it, do so, future realities may be far different from the forecast even though the *statistical* inference was valid.

In general, intention surveys must keep in mind the following limitations:

- How the question is asked can significantly bias the results. For example, the question phrased "Giving blood is essential to the well-being of the community and a duty of all citizens—do you intend to give blood next year?" will probably yield a far higher intention rate than the question "Do you expect to donate blood sometime during the next year?"
- The importance of the choice to the person has a lot to do with whether an intention is carried out. An expressed intention to have a routine physical or be screened for hypertension is less likely to be followed up than an intention to have hernia repair or a sterilization operation.
- Intention to use a familiar service is more likely to be followed than an intention to use an unfamiliar one. Patients at a clinic who say that they will go again are more likely to do so than those expressing an intention to do so for the first time.
- Intentions under the control of the intender are more reliable. A person may express the intention to go to a particular hospital, but that person's physician may not have privileges there or hate the place.
- Intentions that are clearly respected socially and are desirable are likely to be stated more often than followed.
- Intentions that can be carried out immediately or soon are more likely to be followed than those that cannot be carried out for weeks, months, or years.

On the other hand intention surveys can be used to do more than foresee utilization. Respondents may be asked why they intend one way or the other. People expressing their intentions to use a service may be asked to indicate what they expect from it or why they prefer a given provider. People with the opposite intention can be asked to explain their answers and even suggest what might make them change their minds. As the results of the intention survey come in, the organization can take steps to strengthen the good intentions and win over the reluctant respondents.

## SUMMARY

Prospection techniques may be used in a naive manner whenever the dynamics affecting future utilization of health services are felt to be unknowable or too complicated to address. Employment of naive prospection should probably be limited to those circumstances where past utilization data are unavailable and the dynamics affecting future utilization cannot be incorporated.

Delphi is certainly the best-known prospection technique and the most often used. It relies on the consensus of well-informed people as the best insight into the future. In addition to the conventional strict Delphi technique, a variety of modified versions are both possible and frequently used. Various modifications may enhance the extent of group interaction or the type of information employed. Selection of participants is the key to successful Delphi forecasting, though choices may legitimately be made on political as well as technical grounds.

Analogs rely on the tendency of history to repeat itself. If the appropriate past situation can be identified, future utilization may well repeat that situation. Another time in the present place or the present time in another place may be selected as the best analog. Analogs are simple to use once the choice has been made because the totality of past experience—both the level and timing of utilization, for example—should be replicated. The risk is always that the future will not quite repeat the past exactly.

Scenarios rely on properly identifying critical factors whose alternative future states make significant differences to future utilization. By correctly specifying these factors, their potential future states, and the differential effect that such states have on utilization, scenario forecasting can identify probable futures of health services use. If all those alternative states would lead to the same decision, that decision can be made with great confidence. If not, some gamble must be taken, selecting the most probable states, or a commitment made to bringing about the necessary future conditions.

User surveys rely on the ability of people who control or actually use health services to foresee their own behavior. Their ability to do so is subject to a variety of variables, such as the importance of the behavior to them, their familiarity with the type of service to be used, their control over use, the immediacy of the opportunity to follow their intention, and the likelihood of their expressing an intention to please the survey takers. Because surveys are used to identify intention, this approach is also subject to the strengths and limitations of survey research, relative to sample size, representativeness, and inferential confidence.

### Annotated Bibliography

**Ajzen, J., and Fishbein, M.** *Understanding Attitudes and Predicting Social Behavior.* Englewood Cliffs, N.J.: Prentice-Hall, 1980, Chap. 4, pp. 42–52.

Discusses reliability of expressed intentions, noting that when attitudes and subjective values agree with and support intentions; in other words when people can say why they intend to behave in a particular manner, their intentions are more likely to be carried out.

**Bender, A., et al.** "Delphic Study Examines Developments in Medicines." *Future,* June 1969, p. 301.

Describes Delphi forecasting applied to anticipate changes in the technology and practice of medical care.

**Dalkey, N.** *The Delphi Method: An Experimental Study of Group Opinion.* Santa Monica: Rand Corporation, 1969.

A description of the Delphi process as it was developed and used by the Rand Corporation.

**Delbecq, A., et al.** *Group Techniques for Program Planning.* Glenview, IL: Scott Foresman, 1975.

Provides an excellent guide to the use of the Delphi technique.

*Evaluation of Future Hospital Capitalization.* New York: Standard and Poor's Corporation and Booz, Allen & Hamilton, 1978.

Develops three future scenarios of health care utilization based on alternative developments in utilization control efforts, reimbursement, regulation of capital formation, and growth of alternative delivery settings.

**Haglund, K.** "Too Many Doctors." *The New Physician* 27, no. 6 (June 1978): 17.

Discusses what will happen as the probable consequences of a single development, the 57 percent increase in physician–population ratio expected between 1975 and 1990.

*Health Care: Three Reports from 2030 A.D.* Washington, D.C.: Trend Analysis Program, American Council of Life Insurance, 1980.

Includes reports of three groups that addressed what will happen to health care in 50 years.

**Starkweather, D., et al.** "Delphi Forecasting of Health Care Organization." *Inquiry* 12, no. 1 (March 1975): 37.

Describes a nationwide Delphi process used to predict changes in how health services organizations function and are paid.

**Wensley, R.** "Principles of Useful Market Forecasting." *Management Decision* 17, no. 4 (1979): 295.

Argues for usefulness of interactive group processes in forecasting, either on informal basis or through Delphi technique.

# Chapter 13

# Change Factor Forecasting

The change factor approach to forecasting is the prospection counterpart to multivariate techniques used in prediction. It specifically addresses the expected effect of multiple factors taken together. The difference is that both the individual and combined effects of identified change factors are estimated through subjective judgments regarding the future rather than objective analysis based on the past or present.

The change factor technique begins with the identification of change factors to be used. Once identified, the present status of each factor is measured or estimated as accurately as possible together with the present status of whatever utilization is to be forecast. Next the future status of each change factor is individually forecast. Then the possible interactive effects among such factors are estimated, and a revised estimate of the future status of each is developed. Next the expected effect of the forecast change in each factor is estimated.Finally the interactions of the several change factors as they affect utilization are resolved to yield a prospection forecast of future utilization.

## FACTOR IDENTIFICATION

A change factor, for the purpose of this technique, is some characteristic of or some development in the environment that meets the following criteria:

- It has a known or at least confidently estimated effect on the utilization to be forecast.
- That effect is significant rather than barely discernible.
- Its future status can be confidently forecast.
- It is expected to change significantly.

*Known effect* is important because the change factor is to be used in forecasting utilization. If the expected effect of a change in the factor's status cannot be estimated, at least in terms of whether it would have an upward or downward impact, it can't be used in forecasting. This is an unfortunate example of how ignorance can be useful because it limits the number of change factors that must be addressed. It is also a realistic way of limiting the factors because if the effect of a factor cannot be forecast, it is useless in forecasting utilization.

*Significant effect* is another way of limiting the number of factors considered. Unless the known effect is major enough to lead to the belief that a factor will make a difference to the forecast, it makes no sense to include it. One way of thinking about the significance of an effect is to think in terms of the standardized beta used in multiple linear regressions. By what percentage will utilization change for each percentage change in the factor? If the factor must increase a thousand times to increase utilization by 1 percent, its effect is not significant.

*Predictable status* is just as critical as known effect. If a factor has a known, significant impact on utilization but its own future cannot be estimated with any confidence, then it is useless in forecasting utilization. If it could take on two or more discrete or significantly different futures, a scenario approach or contingency forecast could be developed. If its future is truly unpredictable, however, it simply cannot be used.

*Significant change* is important because only a change in the factor could produce a change in utilization. It is helpful to identify important change factors that do not change in order to get a sense of stabilizing influences. Only change factors that change enough to have significant impact on future utilization actually contribute to the forecast, however. It is precisely the estimated amount of change in each factor that is used to forecast the amount of change expected in utilization.

## NOMINAL GROUP TECHNIQUE

A useful technique for identifying change factors is the nominal group technique developed by Delbecq, Van de Ven, and Gustafson. Their book, *Group Techniques for Program Planning: A Guide to Nominal Group and Delphi Processes*, describes this technique in detail as it is applied to planning. Its forte is the development of consensus lists of ideas or items using diverse groups. A useful set of change factors can be identified through use of this technique in one to two hours.

Basically the technique begins with selecting a set of people to participate. They may be selected on the basis of technical knowledge and good judgment or on their political importance in making the decisions to be based on the utilization forecast. For a single group, no more than eight participants should be used, and six is preferable. Multiple groups may be used if larger numbers must be included, requiring a second-order consensus-reaching based on what each individual group comes up with.

The nominal group process begins with explaining the technique to all participants and supplying them with the necessary paper and pencil for each participant and a flip-chart pad or blackboard for each group. All participants are instructed to write as many change factors as appropriate on their individual lists. Given the sorts of factors applicable to utilization of health services, they should be asked to think of change factors in four categories:

1. demographic factors, i.e., objective attributes of populations whose utilization is to be forecast, their size, age mix, proportion covered by insurance, health status, etc.
2. psychographic factors, i.e., subjective attitudes, feelings, and beliefs regarding health and utilization that affect their probability, type, and frequency of use
3. behavioral factors, i.e., the sorts of behavior that influence health status and the need for using health services: smoking, diet, alcohol and drug use, exercise, etc.
4. system factors, i.e., aspects of the general environment and health system that affect health status and utilization: pollution, state of the economy, utilization control efforts by industry, insurance companies and government, etc.

Each person should be given 15 to 20 minutes to prepare a list. No discussion is permitted during this period except for questions addressed to the group leader. Normally participants keep at their task throughout this period, because the group is doing so and there's nothing else to do.

Once the period ends and each participant has a personal list, the group sets out to develop a group list. This is done by asking each participant in turn to nominate one change factor item at a time. Each nomination is simply recorded on the group's flip-chart or blackboard. No discussion is permitted unless the person recording (the group leader in most cases or a selected member if multiple groups are used) doesn't understand or can't spell the factor nominated. No judgment as to the appropriateness of a nomination is permitted until the group list is complete.

Each participant in turn nominates one factor at a time until all the items on each personal list are exhausted. (A round table is best for this process.) This listing process may take 15 to 30 minutes beyond the time to develop each participant's personal list. If the group has spent an hour or so receiving instructions, then carrying out these first two steps, a break would be in order. Normally no break is allowed until after the personal list items have been recorded.

Once the aggregate list is recorded, the group begins judging the items. The change factor selection criteria should be repeated at this stage, and the group asked to consider each nomination in light of these criteria. Some pride of ownership and conflict are likely at this point but shouldn't be serious. Everyone had an equal chance to nominate items, and everyone's items are on the starting list. Even if some are removed, everyone shares in the clarification and selection of the final group list.

Discussion of change factors can take almost any amount of time, depending on how many items were on the original list, how diverse the participants are, and how strong or fragile their egos may be. The group leader should keep discussion focused on the selection criteria and influence the group toward narrowing the list to less than 10 factors. By the time actual forecasts are to be made, 3 to 6 factors are the most workable numbers.

Where people champion unpopular factors, i.e., factors that the rest of the group doesn't understand or agree with, the champion should be given the opportunity to persuade the group. The group leader should direct the champion to explain how the factor works and indicate how much it will change, then how much it will affect utilization. By focusing on specifics, the group can decide whether the factor belongs on the final group list.

The same group that identifies the change factors should in most cases be used to forecast the future of such factors and resolve their impacts. If the nominating group were chosen for political reasons, others may be used to supplement or replace them in the forecasting phase, however. It is entirely a matter of practical judgment which way to go, though using the same group throughout is usually easier and more likely to produce the desired politically or technically sound decision.


## PRESENT STATUS

Once the list of change factors is completed, the present status of each, and the present status of the utilization to be forecast, must be determined. Past data may also be used, with appropriate cautions against relying on observed trends as a substitute for systematic thought and discussion. Present status data are absolutely essential to the change factor approach, however. No one should try to estimate the future of a change factor, and certainly not the future for utilization, without a known starting point. The future is how much the present changes by then.

Ideally the group leader, if a group process is used, anticipates the sort of change factors that the group identifies and has data on the present status of each ready for discussion. Data on present utilization should certainly be available in any case. If the group identifies one or more unexpected change factors, the leader has two choices. The group may be persuaded to delete a factor whose importance is perhaps marginal and for which information is not readily available. Alternatively the group leader can use a lunch hour or other break to acquire the necessary information. Rarely is it possible or desirable to postpone group discussion for days in order to obtain the necessary information, but if that is the only viable choice, so be it.

Whatever aspect of utilization is to be forecast should be thoroughly and accurately measured in the present. This may include volume, user mix, variability, or whatever other attribute of utilization affects the decision. The group members should know from the outset, of course, which attributes are to be forecast as they attempt to identify change factors. Up-to-date, reliable data on the present state of such attributes must then be made available.

## FUTURE STATUS

For each change factor, its future status for the period in which utilization is to be forecast must be identified. Any factors whose future cannot be estimated should have been eliminated earlier. It may be, however, that some factors whose future was thought foreseeable, will not be usable. Either external forecasts or group process may be used at this stage to estimate future status of all change factors to be used.

Some change factors, such as population size, age mix, and location of residences, should be forecast by reliable or at least credible outside agencies. Health department vital statistics sections, electric utilities, councils of governments, universities, or other organizations may be the generally used source of population forecasts in given situations. When external sources of forecasts are available and acceptable for particular change factors, they may be used in preference to group forecasts.

Other factors, however, are likely not to be forecast at all by outside agencies or not to have been forecast reliably or credibly by anyone else. Some may be in the control of or at least subject to the influence of the organization developing the forecast and obviously can't be estimated by anyone else. Others may simply not have been of interest to, or not thought of as predictable by, any other organization. Some change factors probably require internal forecasting.

Where a group is being used for change factor forecasting, which is typically the case, a group process technique such as Delphi (Chapter 12) modified for interaction can be used. Each participant would make an individual prediction. The mean and standard deviation of the group's estimates would be calculated and distributed to members. Each participant could then meditate in silence over subsequent estimates or engage in open discussion to resolve discrepancies. Consensus, voting, or averaging could then be used to develop the group's forecast for the particular factor.

The group should develop as precise and confident a forecast as possible for each change factor's status in the period for which utilization is to be forecast or for a period before that if impacts are known to be time lagged. Precision is especially desirable when multiple change factors are used because any range in future states of change factors is multiplied by the range of other factors in terms of the resulting precision for the utilization forecast. On the other hand, if the best possible estimate for a change factor does cover a considerable range, no attempt should be made to force precision on it artificially.

## FACTOR INTERACTION

Depending on the specific change factors selected, there may be significant interaction among the factors themselves. If two factors chosen are the supply of physicians and charges for a visit, for example, it should be recognized that these affect each other. In the short run a surplus of physicians might conceivably force fees down through competition. Recent experience suggests, however, that a surplus actually forces fees up. Each physician trying to achieve a target income with fewer patients must charge more per encounter. In the long run, if low charges produced low income expectations for physicians, the number of people going into medical school might diminish, thence the supply of physicians decreases.

In effect, change factor approaches can be used to forecast the future of each change factor. Obviously this could lead to perpetual motion forecasting in a backward direction, looking for change factors that affect change factors that affect change factors that affect utilization. It should be recognized, however, that where change factors affect each other as well as utilization, their individual futures should first be applied to each other before they are applied to forecast utilization. In forecasting fees for health services it would simply be poor forecasting not to consider the effect of physician surplus.

**Cross-Impact Matrix**

A relatively simple technique called a *cross-impact matrix* can be helpful in identifying and reflecting the impact of change factors on each other. Each change factor is listed as a column heading and as a row heading in the matrix. At the intersection of each factor with each other factor, an estimate is made first as to whether there is a cross impact, then the direction of that impact, and finally the magnitude of the impact. For each column the sum of the cross impacts is then used to reestimate the future status of the change factor at the head of the column.

In dealing with physician supply and charges for services, for example, a cross-impact matrix would consider the effect of one on the other (Figure 13-1).

Similar cross-impact analysis would be carried out for each change factor. If cross impacts tended in a minus direction for one change factor, that factor's extent of change might be reestimated downward. If all cross impacts were in a plus direction, the future might be reestimated upward. If cross impacts were projected to be a mix of plus and minus effects, a more modest cross-impact effect would probably be expected.

**Expected Effect**

Once the future status of each change factor has been estimated, with appropriate adjustment for cross impacts, the expected effect of changes in each change factor is estimated. The effect of each change factor is first considered individually. Given the expected change in a specific change factor, what effect would it be expected to have on utilization of health services? If physician supply is expected to increase from a ratio of 1 to 750 to a ratio of 1 to 600, what is the effect on utilization of physician services, of hospital services?

**Figure 13-1** Cross-Impact Matrix

|                    |   | Physician Supply        | Charges              |
|--------------------|---|-------------------------|----------------------|
| Physician supply   | – | ✕                       | Short range — plus   |
| Charges            | – | Long range — minus      | ✕                    |
|                    | + | Long range — no change  | ✕                    |

Impact of individual change factors may be estimated objectively or subjectively. For change factors such as age mix, an objective approach is readily available, as suggested in Chapter 9. For factors such as changes in the overall economy or possibly changes in the supply of physicians, a subjective approach may be preferred. Delphi is a particularly appropriate subjective technique for identifying the expected effect of individual change factors. As true for all Delphi approaches, it is advisable to request participants to explain the underlying dynamics that cause them to forecast any specific effect. Other participants can then examine explanatory dynamics as well as the resultant estimate in an objective, critical fashion.

### Interactive Effect

Once the effect of each change factor has been forecast on an individual basis, it is necessary to forecast the combined effect of all such factors, recognizing their interactions. There are basically three ways in which individual factors can relate to each other. They may be totally independent and separate; they may be independent but overlapping; or they may be interdependent and overlapping. Each relationship has a different expected combined effect, so each should be treated differently.

*Independent and separate* effects are additive, each contributing a separate effect regardless of the impact of the other. This is best illustrated by change factors that affect different types of utilization. In forecasting hospital inpatient utilization, for example, change factors that affected surgical admissions would be separate and independent relative to factors that affected only psychiatric or obstetric admissions. An expected increase in ambulatory surgery would be separate and independent from an expected increase in home births in terms of expected impact on hospital utilization.

Where impacts are separate and independent, the best way to deal with them is in terms of absolute numbers or rates. If ambulatory surgery is expected to eliminate 15 admissions per thousand population and home births are expected to eliminate 10 admissions per thousand women aged 15 to 44, their effects should be considered separately and additively. If obstetric admissions were expected to contribute a total of 24 admissions per thousand population, and 4 of these would be eliminated through home births, then the combined effect would be minus 15 for outpatient surgery and minus 4 for home births, equals a combined effect of minus 19.

*Independent and overlapping* effects apply to the same types of utilization and have a multiplicative rather than additive effect. In forecasting utilization of hospital emergency rooms, for example, two change factors might be the growth of immediate care centers (usually called *urgicenters* or *minor emergency centers*) and expected shifts in health insurance coverage requiring deductibles, copayment, or limited coverage of ER visits that don't result in an inpatient admission.

By themselves, each might be projected to have a significant impact. Competition from immediate care centers might be expected to reduce ER utilization 20 percent, for example. Health insurance coverage might be expected to reduce utilization 25 percent. Because the effects of these two factors would be independent but overlapping, their combined effect would not be a decrease of 25 percent + 20 percent = 45 percent. Rather the overlapping nature of their effect would be estimated by percentage impact.

If competition reduces ER utilization 20 percent, then only 80 percent of current ER utilization would remain. If health insurance coverage reduces utilization 25 percent, then only 75 percent of current use would remain. The effect of both change factors, because they are independent but overlapping, would be forecast as .80 × .75 = .60 remaining, or a combined effect of minus 40 percent rather than minus 45 percent.

*Interdependent and overlapping* factors not only affect the same components of utilization but do so in an interdependent way. In other words the effect of one change factor is expected to be greater on the segment of utilization affected by another change factor than on overall utilization as a whole. An example would be estimating the combined effect of growth in ambulatory surgery and increasing implementation of second surgical opinions.

If it is expected that more surgical procedures done on an ambulatory basis would be eliminated by second opinions than would inpatient surgeries, then the combined effect of both change factors would be less than the additive, even less than the multiplicative effect of both. In the extreme case, if all surgeries eliminated by second surgical opinions were also potentially ambulatory, the combined effect of both factors might be no greater than the individual effect of ambulatory surgery alone.

If data are available indicating the extent of interdependence or interaction among specific change factors, then an objective estimate of their interaction would be possible. For example, an analysis of surgery cases being done in hospitals might reveal that 25 percent of all such surgery could be done on an outpatient basis and 25 percent could be eliminated through second surgical opinions. These represent simply the upper bounds of potential impact, not a forecast of probable impact, however.

If 10 percent of all surgeries being done on an inpatient basis are likely to switch to ambulatory, then 10 percent is the expected reduction in surgery cases. If only one-fifth of all surgery patients are likely to seek and be influenced by second opinions, then the expected effect of such a program would be ⅕ × 25 percent, or 5 percent. If the two programs were totally independent, i.e., if they applied to totally distinct subsets of surgery cases, their effect would be additive and their combined effect would be a 15 percent reduction in inpatient surgeries.

If their effects were overlapping, i.e., applied to the same cases but independent, their combined effect would be multiplicative. That is, if the same proportion of ambulatory versus inpatient surgery cases would be eliminated by second opinions, the combined effect would involve some interaction. With 10 percent of all inpatient surgeries eliminated by shifts to ambulatory surgery and 5 percent eliminated through second opinions, the combined effect would be $(100 - 10\%) \times (100 - 5\%) = 85.5\%$ of surgeries remaining or there would be a 14.5% reduction rather than a 15%.

The difference between additive and multiplicative impacts of two factors is likely to be modest but increases with the number of factors. An overlapping and independent set of five factors, each of which contributes a 10% reduction, would have a combined additive impact of 50% but a combined multiplicative impact of $100 - (.9 \times .9 \times .9 \times .9 \times .9) = 41\%$. Similarly five factors each suggesting a 10% increase would produce a combined additive impact of plus 50% but a combined multiplicative impact of $(1.1 \times 1.1 \times 1.1 \times 1.1 \times 1.1) - 100 = +61\%$.

When the surgery change factors are overlapping and independent, something other than an equal proportion of ambulatory cases would be eliminated by second opinions as would inpatient surgery cases. If the ambulatory proportion were less, but greater than zero, the combined effect would be somewhere between the multiplicative and additive effects. If the proportion were greater, up to and including the possibility that *all* the surgery cases would be ambulatory, then the combined effect would be somewhere between the effect of one by itself and the multiplicative effect.

If ambulatory surgery cut out 10 percent of current cases, and of the 5 percent of surgeries expected to be eliminated by second opinions, only one-twentieth were ambulatory, then the combined effect would be 10% + (19/20)(5%) = 14.75%, almost as much as an additive effect. If one-half of all the cases eliminated by second opinions would be ambulatory, then the combined effect would be 10% + (.5)(5%), or 12.5%, less than the 14.5% multiplicative effect. Only when the proportions are independent would the results equal the multiplicative effect, i.e., 10% + (9/10)(5%) = 14.5%, or conversely 5% + (.95)(10%) = 14.5%.

**Multifactor Example**

To illustrate the use of change factor forecasting, consider an attempt to estimate the future rate of inpatient utilization of hospital care in a specified area. To address such a complex challenge, the overall task should first be separated into workable components. This would mean separately identifying the types of inpatient care that make up total utilization: pediatric, obstetric, medical, surgical, and psychiatric. Utilization of these separate categories of service would then be divided into admissions and average length of stay to complete the separation into components.

Each component would be addressed separately insofar as different change factors would tend to affect one differently from others. Ambulatory surgery, for example, would reduce surgical admission rates by eliminating some admissions but would increase length of stay because the eliminated admissions would have been shorter than most others. To address each component, data on present rates would be identified as the starting point. Table 13-1 represents hypothetical component data for illustration. The use rates cannot be added to yield an overall use rate because they apply to different populations. An age-cohort breakdown of the population as in Table 13-2 would produce an overall use rate. Future use rate is then a function of changes in the factors affecting the use of inpatient care by each age and sex cohort plus changes in the proportions that each cohort contributes to the population.

**Table 13-1** Component Utilization Data

| Service Category | Age and Sex Cohort | | Admission Rate | LOS | Use Rate |
|---|---|---|---|---|---|
| Pediatrics | M/F | 0–14 | 50 | 5.0 | 250 |
| Obstetrics | F | 15–44 | 60 | 4.0 | 240 |
| Medicine | M/F | 15+ | 80 | 5.0 | 400 |
| Surgery | M/F | 15+ | 80 | 10.0 | 800 |
| Psychiatric | M/F | 15+ | 10 | 15.0 | 150 |

**Table 13-2** Overall Use Rate

| Service Category | Age and Sex Cohort | | % of Population | × | Cohort-Specific Use Rate | = | Contribution |
|---|---|---|---|---|---|---|---|
| Pediatrics | M/F | 0–14 | 25.0 | | 250 | | 62.5 |
| Obstetrics | F | 15–44 | 20.0 | | 240 | | 48.0 |
| Medicine | M/F | 15+ | 75.0 | | 400 | | 300.0 |
| Surgery | M/F | 15+ | 75.0 | | 800 | | 600.0 |
| Psychiatric | M/F | 15+ | 75.0 | | 160 | | 120.0 |
| | | | | | Total | | 1,130.5 |

Examining just one of these components for illustration, consider obstetric factors. A list of change factors affecting use of inpatient obstetric care by the female population might include the following:

- change factors affecting fertility rates, i.e., the proportion of women, 15 to 44, likely to give birth to babies;
  —age mix within cohort                                           (d)
  —employment and career activities                                (b)
  —family-size preference                                          (p)
  —use of birth control                                            (b)
- change factors affecting the use of inpatient hospital care per birth:
  —preference for nonhospital birth                                (p)
  —cost consciousness                                              (p)
  —health status of mothers                                        (d)
  —health insurance coverage                                       (s)
  —Caesarean deliveries                                            (s)

As true in most cases, this list includes demographic, psychographic, behavior, and system factors, as indicated by the letter in parentheses following each factor listed. As also true of most change factors, those listed are affected by other change factors, such as the state of the economy and social and cultural attitudes. This list illustrates a reasonable set of factors that are direct-impact change factors and might pass the selection criteria in a particular area.

*Age-Mix Effect*

Data on age mix within the 15 to 44 cohort would be obtained from census reports and population forecasts. A shift toward larger proportions in the 30 to 44 end of this cohort would tend to reduce fertility rates because at least historically women in the younger cohorts, especially 20 to 29, are far more likely to bear children in a given year. Age-specific use rates would be used to estimate the expected impact of such a shift. There would presumably be a significant shift, or this factor would not appear on the list. For illustration, let us assume the shift effect in Table 13-3.

Thus the age-mix effect in this case would be predicted to result in a decrease in fertility from 60.0 to 54.0 per thousand, a 10 percent decline. Other change factors may add to or mitigate this decline, of course. This would presumably result in a 10 percent decrease in admissions as well.

**Table 13-3** Shift Effect

| Cohort | Cohort-Specific Fertility Rate | Future Proportion | Contribution |
|--------|-------------------------------|-------------------|--------------|
| 15–19  | 20  | .15 | 3.0 |
| 20–24  | 100 | .15 | 15.0 |
| 25–29  | 120 | .15 | 18.0 |
| 30–34  | 80  | .15 | 12.0 |
| 35–39  | 20  | .20 | 4.0 |
| 40–44  | 10  | .20 | 2.0 |
|        |     |     | 54.0 |

## Employment and Career Effect

If women are expected to be more involved in full-time employment and careers, the expectation would be that they would delay child-rearing and reduce family size, thus diminishing fertility rates. If 50 percent of the female population are in the labor force today and 80 percent are expected to be in the future, then labor force versus non-labor force fertility rates could be used to project the effect. The fertility rate for working women might be 10 per thousand, for example, and that for unemployed women 110 per thousand. Thus, the combined present rate would be $(.50 \times 10) + (.50 \times 110) = 60$. In the future the rate would be $(.80 \times 10) + (.20 \times 110) = 30$. This would suggest a 50 percent reduction in fertility as the employment and career effect.

## Family-Size Preference Effect

For illustration, let us assume that family-size preference amounts to 2.0 children per family with a fertility rate of 60. If preference were to change to 1.5 children per family, we might forecast a reduction in fertility concomitant with the shift in preference, or $(1.5 \div 2.0) \times 60 = 45$. This would suggest a 25 percent reduction in fertility. (At this point it must be noted that the three effects so far examined suggest a decline of 10% + 50% + 25%, which would be 85% if treated additively. These numbers are hypothetical and for illustration only.)

## Birth Control Effect

Just for illustration, let us assume a shift away from birth control pills to a less effective method, due to fear of the health effects of the pill. If the pill were 99 percent effective and the alternative were only 95 percent effective, we would expect an increase of 4 pregnancies per hundred or 40 per thousand. If only 50 percent of the female population were expected to shift from the pill, then the expected effect would be an increase of 20 births per thousand, a 33.3 percent increase over the present rate.

## Nonhospital Preference Effect

For some time roughly 99 percent of all births occur in hospitals. If a dramatic growth in preference for home birth or for alternative birthing centers not part of hospitals were expected, fewer hospital admissions would result. For illustration, let us assume that 5 percent of all women will give birth in places other than hospitals. This would mean a decrease of 4/99 or 4.04 percent in admissions. Length of stay would be expected to increase, say, 1.0 percent, due to elimination of a large number of uncomplicated deliveries.

## Cost-Consciousness Effect

For illustration, let us assume that concern over the high cost of hospital deliveries reduces admissions somewhat but primarily affects length of stay. Admissions might be expected to decline 5 percent but length of stay, 20 percent. Estimates of such effects would be derived through group process discussions and intention surveys.

## Health Status Effect

With growth of concern for health, women might be expected to be better prepared for pregnancy. They might be expected to follow better diet and exercise, reduce smoking, alcohol and drug consumption and be far better prepared physically and mentally for childbirth. This could be taken as the basis for predicting a significant decline in length of stay for each obstetric admission, say, 4.0 to 3.0 days on the average, a 25 percent decline.

## Health Insurance Coverage Effect

Along with other efforts to curb hospital utilization and expenditures, health insurance might be expected to reimburse hospitals a set amount per obstetric delivery. This might tend to reduce length of stay in order to ensure that costs to the hospital per delivery do not exceed the reimbursement. A Delphi process might estimate that length of stay would decline from 4.0 to 3.5 as a result of this factor, a 12.5 percent decline.

*Caesarean Delivery Effect*

With increasing use of fetal monitoring and reduced childbearing per lifetime, there has been an increase in Caesarean over normal deliveries. If the length of stay per Caesarean delivery were 7.0 days, for example, versus normal 3.25, and if 20 percent of deliveries were Caesarean versus 80 percent normal, the current combined length of stay would be

$$
\begin{array}{l}
.20 \times 7.0 \; = 1.4 \\
.80 \times 3.25 = \underline{2.6} \\
\phantom{.80 \times 3.25 = } \underline{4.0}
\end{array}
$$

as indicated earlier. Were the proportion of Caesarean deliveries expected to increase to 40 percent, the expected effect would be

$$
\begin{array}{l}
.40 \times 7.0 \; = 2.8 \\
.60 \times 3.25 = \underline{1.95} \\
\phantom{.60 \times 3.25 = } \underline{4.75}
\end{array}
$$

Thus, average length of stay would be expected to increase by 0.75 days, an 18.75 percent increase from the present 4.0 days.

*Combined Effect*

The individual change factor effects break down as in Table 13-4. For purposes of this illustration, no difference is suggested between fertility and admission rates. As noted, if 99 percent of all births occur in hospitals, there would be a slight difference. Also, there tend to be roughly 1.1 obstetric admissions per live birth, due to false labor, still births, etc. In

**Table 13-4** Individual Change Factor Effects

| Factor | Birth Effect | % | Admission Effect | % | LOS Effect | % |
|---|---|---|---|---|---|---|
| Age mix | − 6.0/1000 | − 10 | − 6.0 | − 10 | | |
| Career | − 30.0/1000 | − 50 | − 30.0 | − 50 | | |
| Family size | − 15.0/1000 | − 25 | − 15.0 | − 25 | | |
| Birth control | + 20.0/1000 | + 33.3 | + 20.0 | + 33.3 | | |
| Nonhospital | | | − 2.4 | − 4.04 | + .04 | + 1.0 |
| Cost consciousness | | | − 3.0 | − 5.0 | | − 20 |
| Health status | | | | | − 1.0 | − 25 |
| Insurance | | | | | − 0.5 | − 12.5 |
| Caesarean | | | | | + 0.75 | + 18.75 |

practice there should be an adjustment for this. In this illustration dealing with percentage changes would reflect admission effects correctly as long as the ratio between live birth and admissions remains constant or is affected only by nonhospital birth preference.

In addressing combined effects, the first step is to determine whether factors are separate and independent, overlapping and independent, or overlapping and interdependent. In going down the list, factors affecting fertility rate alone are presumably independent and separate from those affecting length of stay alone, for example. The factors affecting fertility are potentially overlapping, however, as are all factors affecting length of stay.

Age mix may well be independent of career effect, or larger numbers of career women, might postpone rather than reduce pregnancies and mitigate the age effect. For example, the career effect might greatly increase the age-specific fertility rates in the 30 to 44 segments. If so, the combined effect of career and age-mix change factors would be less than their multiplicative effect. Instead of a 10 percent reduction in admissions due to age mix and a 50 percent reduction due to career effects, suggesting that future admissions would be $.90 \times .50 = .45$ of the present rate, the effects might be totally duplicative, so future admissions would be .50 of the present rate.

Family size might well be a *consequence* of age and career factors rather than separate, in which case it would have no effect of its own. Birth control, however, would presumably be independent of other factors because it represents only a loss in ability to ensure that pregnancies are planned. (Of course, more unplanned pregnancies might lead to an increase in abortions, but this illustration is complicated enough as it is.) Nonhospital births and cost-consciousness effects might also be duplicative if the effect of cost consciousness is to heighten preference for out-of-hospital birth. If so, the total effect of the two factors together would be only the expected effect of the greater, i.e., $-5.0$ percent due to cost consciousness.

Taking into account all factors linked to admissions, there would be a 50 percent reduction in admissions due to the combined effects of age mix, career, and family size. There would be an expected 33.3 percent increase due to birth control ineffectiveness and a 5 percent increase due to cost consciousness. The combined effects of these, if independent of each other, would be that future obstetric admissions should be $.50 \times 1.333 \times .95 = .633$ of the current rate, or 38 per thousand instead of the present 60.

With length of stay, nonhospital birth effects and cost-consciousness effects would be independent. The former results from a reduction in short-stay admissions while the latter applies to hospital admissions. Health status might interact with cost consciousness if younger women tend to be both healthier and more cost conscious, for example. Their combined effect might be somewhere between the .80 × .75 = .60, i.e., a 40 percent reduction expected if independent and the 25 percent reduction expected if totally duplicative. For illustration, say that the combined effect is a 35 percent reduction. The insurance effect might be totally duplicated in the cost-consciousness effect while the Caesarean effect should be independent.

With all factors affecting length of stay together, there would be a 1.0 percent increase expected from home births, a 35 percent reduction from the combination of health status and cost consciousness, no separate effect from insurance, and an increase of 18.75 percent from increased numbers of Caesarean deliveries. The combined effects of all these should be that expected length of stay for obstetrics will be 1.01 × .65 × 1.1875 = .7796 of the present 4.0, or 3.118 days. The future obstetrics use rate would then be 38 × 3.118 = 118.50 patient days per thousand rather than the 60 × 4.0 = 240 at present. The same result would be obtained by multiplying all change factor effects together:

$$.50 \times 1.333 \times .95 \times 1.01 \times .65 \times 1.1875 = .4937$$
$$.4937 \times 240 = 118.50 \text{ patient days per thousand}$$

In most cases the number of significant change factors is less than the nine factors used in this illustration. However many factors, the process of estimating individual and combined effects still enables the development of a forecast based on as many as can be considered. Where quantitative analytical techniques and objective forecasts are not available, the change factor approach at least permits addressing complex causal dynamics.

## SUMMARY

A change factor approach to forecasting use of health services employs subjective estimates of future developments and their impact in a multivariate manner, similar to the way the multiple linear regression performs with objective analysis. It begins with a careful identification of change factors, based on their known, significant impact on health services use and their foreseeable likelihood of significant change. A group process approach such as the nominal group technique can be useful in this identification.

Change factors are first studied to determine their present status, then estimated as to their probable future status, using a subjective process such as Delphi. The impact of their status changes over time is then considered, perhaps using a technique like the cross-impact matrix. The effects of specific factor changes are considered in terms of their independent and separate or overlapping impacts on health services use.

Although this is a subjective approach, it employs specific mathematical estimates of effect and estimates the interacting impact on health services utilization in a quantitative manner. As a consequence it directly produces a quantitative estimate of utilization just as a Delphi process does. It differs from the Delphi approach in explicitly addressing the reasons for anticipated changes.

**Annotated Bibliography**

**Delbecq, A., et al.** *Group Techniques for Program Planning.* Glenview, Ill.: Scott Foresman, 1975.
  Provides an excellent description of how to use a nominal group technique by the developers of this technique.

**Goldsmith, J.** *Can Hospitals Survive?* Homewood, Ill.: Dow-Jones–Irwin, 1981, p. 16.
  Predicts decline in inpatient demand based on developments in a series of change factors whose future direction is foreseeable.

**Harrington, M.** "Forecasting Areawide Demand for Health Care Services: A Critical Review of Major Techniques and Their Application." *Inquiry* 14, no. 3 (September 1977): 254.
  Discusses the factors that affect demand for health services and the impacts that system changes would have on future demand.

**Harris, J.** "Computer Modeling Helps Decision Makers." *Hospital Financial Management* 36, no. 6 (June 1982): 10.
  Describes a computer modeling approach to change factor forecasting, permitting interactive use of such factors to evaluate capital expenditure consequences of future utilization.

**Martino, J.** "Technological Forecasting—An Overview." *Management Science* 26, no. 1 (January 1980): 28.
  Describes subjective techniques for estimating the impact of changes, including the cross-impact matrix.

**Mitchell, F.** "Anticipation versus Results: An Approach to Improved Program Forecasting." *American Journal of Health Planning* 1, no. 2 (April 1978): 7.
  Discusses the elements of the change process in health care and the "mental model" most commonly used in forecasting.

**Pekarna, D., et al.** "Population and Diagnosis-Based Model Projects Bed Needs." *Hospital Progress* 63, no. 1 (January 1982): 52.
  Describes a computer software package called AUTOGRP, which was used to estimate impact of change factors on utilization by diagnosis in hospitals.

# Part V

# Utilization Fluctuations

In many cases, it is not merely the total volume of utilization that has to be forecast in order to make an effective decision. The fluctuations in utilization that might be expected, from hour to hour, day to day, week to week, month to month, and year to year may be important determinants of success for particular decisions. Budgeting, staffing decisions, ordering of supplies, and many other management decisions must anticipate short-term fluctuations in utilization. Decisions regarding whether, when, and by how much to modify structural capacities to accommodate utilization will usually require anticipation of year to year changes in utilization.

There are three principal approaches to forecasting fluctuations in utilization. The simplest, used primarily for anticipating short-term variations, identifies patterns through calculation of ratios. A second approach uses geometric functions to calculate repeating cycles that may be present. The third employs statistical models to predict patterns of fluctuation, with particular emphasis on extreme levels of utilization above the norm.

Chapter 14 addresses patterns of utilization variations found within a given year. Simple mathematics can be used to identify regular patterns in hour to hour, day to day, week to week, and month to month fluctuations. Fourier regression analysis can be used to identify repeating cycles, if they conform to sinusoidal wave forms. A special adaptation of the normal statistical distribution, based on a synthetic standard deviation, will be used to forecast peak utilization levels in hospital inpatient units.

Chapter 15 deals with year to year fluctuations in utilization. Such fluctuations are primarily of concern in planning inpatient capacity changes, but are also useful in forecasting occupancy expectations. The reality of changing annual utilization levels is also important to most other health service providers, however. It is just that with hospitals, the consequences are most serious and least recognized. A model called order statistics will be used to predict patterns of annual fluctuation, with special emphasis on forecasting highest years of utilization.

Chapter 16 identifies a technique that uses known patterns of variation in census to develop early warning re-estimates of utilization, based on additional experience following original forecasts. The consistency of past variations is often quite high, and can be used to reassess forecasts of immediate and intermediate-term utilization, in order to maximize decision flexibility and effectiveness. In effect, this technique serves to verify or cast doubt on original forecasts and their corresponding decisions.

The importance and impact of both random and deliberate fluctuations in utilization have rarely been fully identified or appreciated. The public, abetted by criticisms of various policy analysts, may believe that the capacity of the health care system is clearly excessive, as evidenced by less than 100 percent occupancy of hospitals, for example. Yet surely anyone familiar with fixed capacity and production is aware that 100 percent capacity use is rarely if ever achieved, much less maintained. Hotels, airlines, public and private buildings of all types have to operate so as to survive on far less than 100 percent occupancy; only prisons enjoy continued full occupancy. Barbers, banks, restaurants, and all other service industries would be flabbergasted if they averaged anything close to 100 percent use of their capacities, and would be striving to increase capacity should such use occur.

The patterns of variability that will be described in Chapters 14 and 15 seem to be inevitable and universal. They indicate that smaller-volume providers can expect greater fluctuations in utilization, both year-to-year and day-to-day, than larger-volume providers. This tends to add to the economies of scale for larger providers, but undermines the viability of smaller. Rural areas, small hospitals, solo practitioners, all must face this discomfiting reality.

More important, perhaps, are the implications of such variability for public policy. Any attempt by government, industry, or insurance organizations to set uniform payment levels for all services, or enforce uniform occupancy levels for all hospitals, flies in the face of inescapable, statistical realities. It may seem, on the face, to be eminently proper and just to treat all providers and services equally, i.e. not to discriminate based on size or location. Given the fact that utilization experience will be inescapably different depending on the volume of use, however, it would seem both proper and necessary to discriminate, i.e. to recognize such differences and reflect them in public policy and payment.

# Chapter 14

# Utilization Fluctuations within the Year

The variability of utilization within the year is an unavoidable and significant fact of life for virtually all providers of health care. Emergency room and immediate care programs (urgicenters, walk-in clinics, etc.) experience substantial variations in demand from hour to hour every day. Day-of-the-week fluctuation patterns characterize admissions to hospitals as well as emergency care demand, with particularly serious trauma more common on week-end and payday evenings. Seasonal fluctuations in demand may relate to cold and flu increases in the winter, ski injuries or drownings in resort areas by season. Hunting seasons may produce dramatic increases in poison ivy cases, gunshot wounds, or other injuries.

To the extent that such fluctuations may be consistent, and linked to known factors in the environment, they may be predictable. To the extent that they can be accurately forecast, they can enable appropriate management and short-term planning decisions. In practice short-term fluctuations in utilization can often be predicted with greater accuracy than long-term volumes.

Three different approaches may be used to predict short-term fluctuations in utilization. The simplest expresses hourly, daily and seasonal fluctuation patterns as functions of consistent mathematical relationships. Ratios are calculated between the underlying mean or trend in overall utilization and the use of services in specific hours, days, weeks, or months. A slightly more complex approach looks for cycles of consistent frequency and amplitude within the year. A third technique employs the normal statistical distribution to predict peak utilization levels within a given year.

## RATIO TECHNIQUES

The mathematical relationship between utilization in a short period and a longer period can be expressed as a ratio. This can be done in a number

189

of ways, but the most useful are probably the *part-to-whole* ratio and the *relative average* ratio. If such ratios are consistent enough over time or space and are expected to be persistent as well, they can be used to predict utilization levels for specific periods in the future.

*Part-to-whole* ratios calculate the relationship between utilization of services in one unit of time to utilization in a larger unit of which it is usually a part. If total daily utilization in an immediate care center were 50 visits, for example, and it were open for 12 hours in the day, each hour would be theoretically expected to see one-twelfth or 8.33 percent of daily volumes per hour. In practice, however, hourly patterns might look more like the data in Table 14-1.

In knowing that such patterns are typically the case and confidently expecting their persistence, appropriate planning and management decisions could be made. Special lunch-hour assignments could be made to ensure adequate coverage during the noon–2:00 P.M. period when utilization is high. Staffing could be arranged to involve light coverage from 9:00 A.M.–noon, then starting additional staff at noon. If early staff would end their shifts at 5:00 P.M., part-time staff might be used to cover heavy-use hours in the evening.

For that matter, hours could actually be changed in hopes of attracting more total volume per day. With low use in the early morning, the center might decide to open from 10:00 A.M.–10:00 P.M. in hopes that utilization in the new 9:00–9:59 P.M. period would be greater than in the old 9:00–9:59 A.M. period. The center might open at 11:00 A.M. or even noon and

**Table 14-1** Hourly Patterns

| Period | Mean % of Daily Volume | Mean Visits per Period |
|---|---|---|
| 9:00– 9:59 A.M. | 4.2 | 2.1 |
| 10:00–10:59 A.M. | 5.4 | 2.7 |
| 11:00–11:59 A.M. | 6.8 | 3.4 |
| 12:00–12:59 P.M. | 12.4 | 6.2 |
| 1:00– 1:59 P.M. | 9.6 | 4.8 |
| 2:00– 2:59 P.M. | 6.2 | 3.1 |
| 3:00– 3:59 P.M. | 4.4 | 2.2 |
| 4:00– 4:59 P.M. | 6.2 | 3.1 |
| 5:00– 5:59 P.M. | 10.6 | 5.3 |
| 6:00– 6:59 P.M. | 12.2 | 6.1 |
| 7:00– 7:59 P.M. | 13.0 | 6.5 |
| 8:00– 8:59 P.M. | 9.0 | 4.5 |
| Total | 100.0 | 50.0 |

take advantage of cost savings for staff even though expecting fewer total visits per day.

Day-of-the-week fluctuation might follow a consistent pattern, as do admissions to hospitals, especially for elective surgery. Such admissions are characterized by high numbers on Sunday, Monday, and Tuesday afternoons, then declining numbers on Wednesday, Thursday, and Friday, down to practically none on Saturday. (Special efforts might be made to smooth out such patterns, especially if surgery operates six or seven days per week rather than five.)

A typical pattern might look like Table 14-2. If total predicted admissions for the week were 30, expected admissions for each day could be predicted based on the mean proportions for each day in the past. Daily census for each day could be predicted based on predicted discharges of patients already in the hospital, then the predicted daily admissions and length of stay for new patients. Staffing levels in admitting departments could be arranged to mirror expected variability in daily admissions.

Within the year, utilization from week to week and month to month might follow similar patterns. Inpatient census, for example, tends to be high during the winter and low in the summer, with precipitous drop-off during the Christmas to New Year period. Obstetric utilization seems to peak around March to April, decline in the summer, rise again in October, then drop again during the winter. Pediatric census varies more than other services and is affected by the timing of school holidays and the beginning and end of school. Psychiatric census tends to vary more randomly but may increase around family stress periods, including holidays.

Expressing each month's utilization as a percentage of the total utilization for the year might produce a pattern such as in Table 14-3. Some variations in utilization per month would be expected from the fact that months have different numbers of days. As Table 14-3 indicates, however,

**Table 14-2** Fluctuation Pattern

| Day | Mean Admissions/Day | % of Weekly Admissions |
|---|---|---|
| Monday | 11.2 | 32.0 |
| Tuesday | 9.1 | 26.0 |
| Wednesday | 3.4 | 9.7 |
| Thursday | 2.4 | 6.9 |
| Friday | 1.7 | 4.9 |
| Saturday | 0.2 | 0.6 |
| Sunday | 7.0 | 20.0 |
| Total | 35.0 | 100.1 |

**Table 14-3** Monthly Utilization Pattern

| Month | % of Year's Days | % of Year's Utilization |
|---|---|---|
| January | 8.49 | 9.46 |
| February | 7.67 | 8.67 |
| March | 8.49 | 9.51 |
| April | 8.22 | 8.36 |
| May | 8.49 | 8.45 |
| June | 8.22 | 8.01 |
| July | 8.49 | 7.33 |
| August | 8.49 | 7.28 |
| September | 8.22 | 7.87 |
| October | 8.49 | 8.75 |
| November | 8.22 | 8.36 |
| December | 8.49 | 7.95 |
| Totals | 99.98 | 100.00 |

some seasonal factors have a greater effect than the day count. If such ratios have been consistent and are expected to be persistent, the expected utilization for each month could be predicted once a year's utilization is forecast. With monthly utilization predictions, purchasing of food, staffing decisions, vacation timing, etc., can be handled more efficiently.

**RELATIVE RATIOS**

Another approach to expressing the same patterns is to calculate average utilization for each component period and then for the entire period. Each component's average could then be expressed as a ratio to the overall average. Hour-of-the-day utilization, expressed earlier as proportions of the whole, would look like the data in Table 14-4 if expressed as relative ratios.

The ratios to the mean clearly indicate how much variability in utilization there is from hour to hour. It ranges from as low as half the mean volume to over one-and-one-half times the mean volume, i.e., with a factor of three. This could be directly translated into staffing patterns more readily than component percentages. It takes only a little more time to calculate ratios to the mean, so where better decisions or even easier decisions would result, the relative averages should be used.

A similar analysis of daily admissions, employing the same data as the component percentage analysis, would yield the data in Table 14-5. Here again the relation to the mean gives a clearer picture of the variation pattern. Extreme differences are apparent, from 2.24 times the average

**Table 14-4** Hour-of-the-Day Utilization

| Period | Volume per Hour | Ratio to Mean |
|---|---|---|
| 9:00– 9:59 A.M. | 2.1 | .504 |
| 10:00–10:59 A.M. | 2.7 | .647 |
| 11:00–11:59 A.M. | 3.4 | .815 |
| 12:00–12:59 P.M. | 6.2 | 1.487 |
| 1:00– 1:59 P.M. | 4.8 | 1.151 |
| 2:00– 2:59 P.M. | 3.1 | .743 |
| 3:00– 3:59 P.M. | 2.2 | .528 |
| 4:00– 4:59 P.M. | 3.1 | .743 |
| 5:00– 5:59 P.M. | 5.3 | 1.271 |
| 6:00– 6:59 P.M. | 6.1 | 1.463 |
| 7:00– 7:59 P.M. | 6.5 | 1.559 |
| 8:00– 8:59 P.M. | 4.5 | 1.079 |
| Mean | 4.17 | |

**Table 14-5** Daily Admissions Relative to Mean

| Day | Mean Admissions per Day | Ratio to Weekly Mean |
|---|---|---|
| Monday | 11.2 | 2.24 |
| Tuesday | 9.1 | 1.82 |
| Wednesday | 3.4 | 0.68 |
| Thursday | 2.4 | 0.48 |
| Friday | 1.7 | 0.34 |
| Saturday | 0.2 | 0.04 |
| Sunday | 7.0 | 1.40 |
| Weekly mean | 5.0 | |

admission load to only 4 percent of the average, a 56-times difference. It is unlikely that staffing would be adjusted to conform exactly to these extremes, though use of part-time personnel could result in greater efficiency for the admitting department.

For seasonal patterns relative ratios might look something like Table 14-6.

## PATTERN COMBINATIONS

With multiple fluctuation patterns apparent in utilization of health services, they can be used to forecast expected utilization for any specific period. In order to predict the census on a given day of the year, for example, we could start with the forecast that the year's utilization will

**Table 14-6** Seasonal Patterns

| Month | Monthly ADC | Relative Ratio |
|---|---|---|
| January | 139.3 | 1.114 |
| February | 141.3 | 1.130 |
| March | 140.0 | 1.120 |
| April | 127.1 | 1.017 |
| May | 124.4 | .995 |
| June | 121.8 | .974 |
| July | 107.9 | .863 |
| August | 107.2 | .857 |
| September | 119.7 | .957 |
| October | 128.8 | 1.031 |
| November | 127.1 | 1.017 |
| December | 117.0 | .936 |
| Year's ADC = | 125 | |

amount to 36,500 patient visits, 100 per day (or patient days, services, or whatever is being forecast). If the day to be forecast is a Tuesday in the third week of March, we would first note that March has a ratio of 112 percent of the year's average. The third week in March might have a ratio of 104 percent of the March average. Tuesday might have a ratio of 122 percent of the week's average. If so, the expected number of visits on that Tuesday would be 112% × 104% × 122% × 100 visits, or 142 visits.

The value of using relative ratios is even more apparent when combining variability patterns. Relative ratios can simply be multiplied by each other to yield the combined prediction. Without such ratios, separate calculations would have to be made for each step.

Patterns of variability may vary from year to year. March utilization, for example, may have ranged from 1.02 times the year's average to 1.22, with an average of 1.12. If the average ratio is used as the best guess for a future March, it must be recognized that future ratios could easily be 1.02, 1.22, or anything between and still be consistent with past experience. If such a range produces too great an uncertainty or lack of precision in a forecast, it simply reflects a lack of consistency in the past.

Using observed patterns of hourly, daily, weekly, or monthly utilization fluctuations to predict utilization depends on the persistence as well as consistency of such patterns. The more consistent patterns have been in the past, the more precise forecasts of the future based on them will be. Less consistent patterns necessarily result in less precise forecasts.

Persistence is a more critical problem because the basic prediction approach depends on the continuation of past patterns. As with all prediction techniques, it is best to look for the causal dynamics responsible for the pattern. If those dynamics are identified and understood and if there is sound reasoning to believe that they will operate essentially the same in the future, then relying on the pattern for prediction is at least reasonable.

## Cycles

Hourly patterns that are repeated every day are cycles, as are daily patterns repeated every week, weekly patterns repeated every month, and monthly patterns repeated every year. There may, however, be patterns that don't conform exactly to hourly, daily, weekly, or monthly units. Also cyclical analysis can provide measures of the consistency in past relationships to aid in judging whether to rely on them in forecasting.

A particular type of regression, called a *Fourier regression*, specifically incorporates a sinusoidal wave cycle. This is a cycle of consistent length and amplitude, with symmetrical deviations both above and below the "line" representing the mean, i.e., expected value for the larger period, or a linear trend if one is present. The form of this regression is complicated but not beyond the capacity of modern handheld calculators.

The Fourier regression takes the form

$$y = a + b_1 t + b_2 \sin \frac{2\pi t}{L} + b_3 \cos \frac{2\pi t}{L}$$

where $y$ = utilization
$b_1$, $b_2$, and $b_3$ = coefficients
$t$ = time, e.g., days, weeks, months, years
$L$ = number of units of time in each cycle

Sine and cosine can be calculated easily on most scientific calculators. With the basic Fourier formula, past utilization can be analyzed to determine if any regular cycle characterizes past experience.

In effect the Fourier regression is a multiple linear regression with three independent variables. Because it is a time series model, it requires many years of utilization data from the same situation; cross-sectional analysis of multiple situations over the same time frame doesn't apply. An absolute minimum of one cycle *(L)* is required to employ a Fourier analysis. Ideally more than one cycle should be available to ensure that a regular, persistent cycle has been identified rather than a one-time situation.

## FLUCTUATION PREDICTIONS

The forecasting of regular fluctuations in utilization is a prediction process because it predicates specific utilization levels on some underlying expected value for a larger period. Predicting visits per hour in a given day applies past relationships between hourly and total daily utilization to a forecast of utilization for a given day. Predicting seasonal fluctuations in monthly hospital census would multiply monthly ratios times an expected annual utilization level. Predicting cyclical variations in utilization employs a calculated cycle pattern applied to an underlying trend in year-to-year utilization.

The prediction of fluctuations is important when and because a specific decision has to be made based on the utilization for a specific short period within the longer period. Staffing decisions or choices of the number of chairs in the waiting room might be geared to the peak number of visits expected in a given hour of the day or day of the week, for example. Staffing levels and vacation timing might be geared to the expected peak and low months of hospital utilization. The bed capacity of a hospital might be determined based on yearly cyclical fluctuations around a long-term trend (see Chapter 15).

**Example 1**

Table 14-7 shows hourly visits in an immediate care center where daily visits are expected to be 60.

**Table 14-7** Hourly Visits

| Hourly Period | Mean Past % of Daily Visits × 60 = | Expected Number of Visits |
|---|---|---|
| 9:00– 9:59 A.M. | 4.2 | 2.5 |
| 10:00–10:59 A.M. | 5.4 | 3.2 |
| 11:00–11:59 A.M. | 6.8 | 4.1 |
| 12:00–12:59 P.M. | 12.4 | 7.4 |
| 1:00– 1:59 P.M. | 9.6 | 5.8 |
| 2:00– 2:59 P.M. | 6.2 | 3.7 |
| 3:00– 3:59 P.M. | 4.4 | 2.6 |
| 4:00– 4:59 P.M. | 6.2 | 3.7 |
| 5:00– 5:59 P.M. | 10.6 | 6.4 |
| 6:00– 6:59 P.M. | 12.2 | 7.3 |
| 7:00– 7:59 P.M. | 13.0 | 7.8 |
| 8:00– 8:59 P.M. | 9.0 | 5.4 |
| | 100.0 | 59.9 |

**Example 2**

Table 14-8 shows daily visits to the immediate care center where the weekly volume is expected to be 400.

**Example 3**

Table 14-9 shows monthly average daily census (ADC) during a year when hospital ADC equals 125. In order to predict the specific utilization volume for a given hour, the year's utilization might first be forecast. Then the utilization for a given month could be predicted based on monthly variation patterns. If there are no consistent weekly variation patterns

**Table 14-8** Daily Visits

| Period | Past % of Weekly Visits × 400 = | Expected Number of Daily Visits |
|---|---|---|
| Monday | 16 | 64 |
| Tuesday | 14 | 56 |
| Wednesday | 18 | 72 |
| Thursday | 17 | 68 |
| Friday | 20 | 80 |
| Saturday | 15 | 60 |
| | 100 | 400 |

**Table 14-9** Monthly ADC

| Month | Past Proportion of Patient Days × | Year's Patient Days (125 × 365) | Expected Month's = Patient Days ÷ | Days in Month = | Monthly ADC |
|---|---|---|---|---|---|
| Jan. | .0946 | | 4,316 | 31 | 139.2 |
| Feb. | .0867 | | 3,956 | 28 | 141.3 |
| Mar. | .0949 | | 4,330 | 31 | 139.7 |
| Apr. | .0838 | | 3,823 | 30 | 127.4 |
| May | .0845 | | 3,855 | 31 | 124.4 |
| June | .0801 | | 3,655 | 30 | 121.8 |
| July | .0733 | | 3,344 | 31 | 107.9 |
| Aug. | .0728 | | 3,322 | 31 | 107.2 |
| Sep. | .0787 | | 3,591 | 30 | 119.7 |
| Oct. | .0875 | | 3,992 | 31 | 128.8 |
| Nov. | .0836 | | 3,814 | 30 | 127.1 |
| Dec. | .0795 | | 3,627 | 31 | 117.0 |
| | 1.0000 | | 45,625 | 365 | 125 |

within a month, the utilization for a week would be predicted as a proportion of the whole month, e.g., 25 percent for February, less for other months (adjusting for weekends). With a weekly forecast, utilization for a given day could be predicted based on daily fluctuations within the week, and hourly utilization based on patterns of hourly fluctuations.

**Fluctuation Patterns**

Often it is not the utilization for a specific hour, day, week, or month that is to be forecast but the overall pattern for an entire year. In such cases the full density function or distribution of utilization levels must be forecast. For example, the staffing level of a hospital might be planned based on expected peak daily census levels within the year. Under such circumstances the task would be to forecast the highest expected daily census levels given the yearly utilization forecast.

**SYNTHETIC STANDARD DEVIATION**

The Gaussian or normal statistical distribution has been used for more than 35 years as a model for the annual variability of daily inpatient census in hospitals. The advantage of this model lies in its ability to predict the extent and frequency of daily census levels above the mean or average daily census. Armed with such a predictive model, planners and administrators can discuss total bed needs in light of the likelihood or expected frequency of days in which all available beds would be filled.

The model works with admirable simplicity. Once the ADC of a hospital is predicted, its standard deviation is usually estimated as the square root of ADC. This square root model is based on the Poisson-Normal approximation, in which the variance equals the mean (from Poisson); hence the standard deviation equals the square root of the mean. Once the standard deviation is known (or estimated), any bed capacity under consideration can be translated into a protection level.

The protection level is the proportion of the time that the daily census would be expected to be less than the bed capacity. This is the complement of the turnaway rate, or proportion of the time that all beds would be expected to be filled. A capacity equal to 2.327 standard deviations above the mean (ADC) should be completely filled only 1.0 percent of the time, hence represents 99 percent protection. A standby capacity equal to 2.054 standard deviations represents 98 percent protection; one equal to 1.645 standard deviations represents 95 percent protection.

Three rather damning problems attend this approach, however, despite its long history. First, the daily census in hospitals does not appear to conform particularly well to the normal distribution model. Second, the actual standard deviation of the daily census tends significantly and consistently to exceed the square root of ADC when it is calculated from empirical data. Third, when the true, calculated standard deviation is employed with the normal distribution model, it tends to exaggerate bed needs.

**Nonconforming Annual Census**

The actual pattern of daily census for a full year in a hospital is likely to be significantly at variance with the normal distribution. The familiar bell-shaped curve would expect the frequency of daily census to be portrayed graphically (Figure 14-1). Based on examination of over 300 cases from eight states, actual daily census distributions tend to follow one of the forms in Figures 14-2 through 14-5.

When the ADC level is small, especially when less than 10, the daily census cannot evidence the expected lower or left-hand "tail" of the normal distribution because it cannot go below a value of zero (Figure 14-2). When the capacity of the hospital cannot be stretched to the expected peak daily census levels, the census distribution becomes truncated by running out of beds, hence loses its upper or right-hand "tail" (Figures 14-3 and 14-5). When the average daily census is larger, i.e., above 16, the extremely low occupancy that prevails during the Christmas to New Year

**Figure 14-1** Frequency of Daily Census

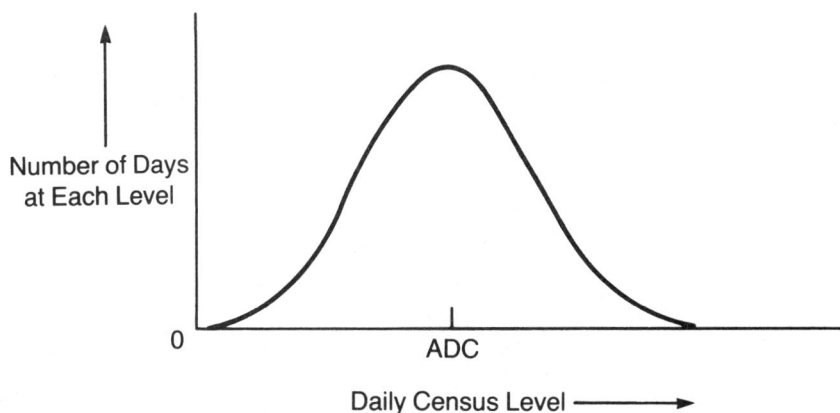

**Figure 14-2** Typical Poisson—Small ADC

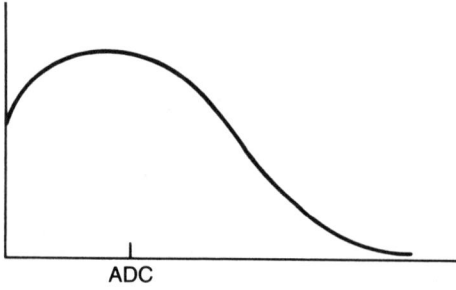

ADC

**Figure 14-3** Truncated Poisson—Small ADC Inadequate Beds

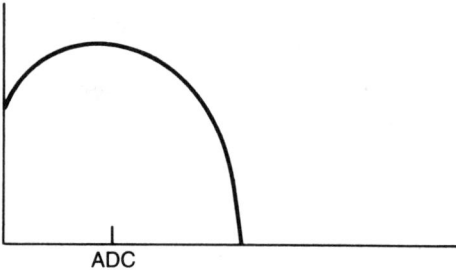

ADC

**Figure 14-4** Skewed Normal—Larger ADC (>16)

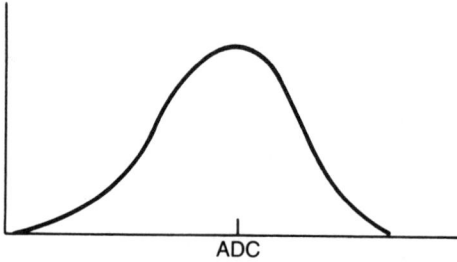

ADC

**Figure 14-5** Truncated Normal—Larger ADC Inadequate Beds

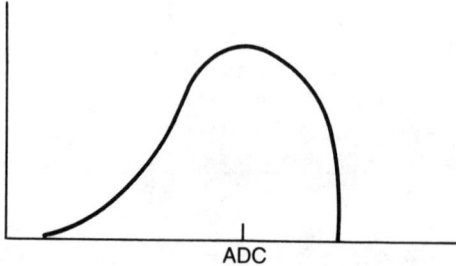

ADC

period extends the left-hand tail and makes the distribution asymmetrical. The lowest day is typically farther away from the mean (ADC) than the highest census day.

Moreover for nontruncated distributions (Figure 14-4) there tends to be greater dispersion around the mean of ADC than is expected in the normal distribution. There is a lower frequency of days close to the ADC and a greater frequency of days away from the ADC than is characteristic of the normal distribution. Graphically speaking, the actual census distribution differs from the expected, as shown in Figure 14-6.

The probability that actual daily census patterns would not conform to the normal distribution model has long been recognized. The conditions for such a random or stochastic distribution (independent, "natural" events) simply do not hold for hospital utilization except perhaps for obstetrics or intensive and coronary care units. It has generally been felt, however, that the normal distribution comes close enough to make it useful. It is entirely a matter of judgment, of course, as to how close is close enough. To judge the risk in adopting the normal distribution model as an approximation, it is necessary to examine both the estimate of standard deviation typically employed and actual standard deviations.

**Untenable Square Root Estimate**

The fact that the square root of the ADC is not a perfect estimate of the standard deviation has been known for some time. When the standard deviation for a full year's daily census figures is calculated, it consistently comes out above the square root of ADC to a degree that increases as the size of the ADC increases. Based on examination of 300 hospital-years of

**Figure 14-6** Actual Census Distribution

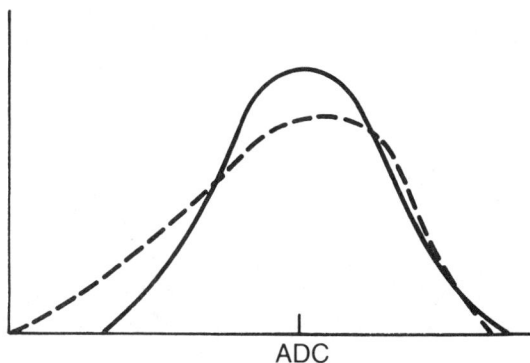

ADC

data from eight states, the actual standard deviation is roughly 10 percent higher than the square root of ADC when ADC is about 15, roughly 20 percent higher when ADC is about 50, roughly 50 percent higher when ADC is about 150, roughly 75 percent higher when ADC is about 250, and roughly 100 percent higher or twice the square root of ADC when ADC is about 500. For clusters of hospitals, where aggregate ADC may be well into the thousands, the discrepancy between predicted and actual standard deviation becomes far worse. For a cluster with an ADC of 3,050, for example, the calculated standard deviation was over 250, while the square root of 3,050 is only 55.2.

As long as issues being discussed relate to the variability of the daily census in small units, the discrepancy between observed and actual standard deviations need not have catastrophic consequences. As the size of the ADC increases, however, the extent to which the square root of ADC estimate is good enough comes increasingly in doubt. Although plus or minus 10 percent or even 20 percent might seem close enough, the estimating model seems hardly tenable where actual values are half again or twice as large as expected and more.

**Untenable Actual Standard Deviation**

Yet a third disappointment awaits in attempting to use the empirically derived standard deviation to estimate protection or turnaway levels and thereby determine bed needs. If the actual standard deviation value is plugged into the normal distribution table, protection levels thus derived tend to be exaggerated significantly. For a hospital with an ADC of 150, for example, observed standard deviations averaged roughly 18.0. To achieve a 99 percent protection should require a standby capacity of 2.33 $\times$ 18 = 42 beds, for a total of 192 beds. In reality such a protection level could be achieved with a 35-bed standby capacity, or a total of 186 beds.

In work carried out independently from the author's analysis, essentially the same results have been found. Cowen found, for example, that a hospital with an ADC of 192.3 had an actual standard deviation of 24.8 (compared to a square root of ADC equal to 13.9). This would suggest a 99 percent protection level at 192.3 + 2.33(24.8) = 250.1, whereas such a protection level was actually achieved at 239.5 (see bibliography).

This finding is understandable considering the fact that actual daily census does not fit the normal distribution model well. Because low or "left-tail" values are skewed far below expected levels by Christmas and because the overall distribution is more scattered around the mean, hence "flatter" than expected, calculated standard deviations tend to be high. These exaggerated standard deviations then estimate higher than actual peak daily census levels, hence exaggerate the bed needs required to achieve specific protection levels.

Because the observed standard deviation greatly overstates the extent and frequency of peak daily census levels, the traditional square root of ADC estimate might do a better job. This is not the case. When applied specifically to the task of estimating the top daily census levels, the square root of ADC, used with normal distribution table values, consistently understates peak census levels. For small ADC levels, the degree of understatement is small, but the error increases significantly with increasing ADC levels. For an ADC of 25, for example, the theoretical 99 percent protection level would be $25 + 2.33(\sqrt{25}) = 36.65$; the actual value is 38. For an ADC of 100, the theoretical value would be 123.3; the actual is 129. For an ADC of 400, the theoretical value would be 446.6, while the actual value is 461.

As a general rule the observed standard deviation significantly overstates the number of beds needed to achieve any selected protection level, hence exaggerates capacity requirements for any year. The square root model in contrast significantly understates the capacity necessary for a given protection level and more so for larger hospitals than for smaller. The amount of over and understatement by these alternative models tends to be significant, especially for larger hospitals or clusters of institutions.

**The Synthetic Standard Deviation**

A way out of the dilemma created by these discomfiting findings is suggested by focusing on the essential purpose of using *any* statistical distribution model. That purpose is to predict the extent and frequency of a relatively small number of daily census levels, given the mean or ADC. A useful model is not required to predict accurately the extent and frequency of *all* daily census levels. Those below the mean and even those close to the mean are of no particular account in discussing bed or capacity requirements. It is customary to determine bed needs based on protection levels that range no lower than 95 percent, that usually cluster around 98 to 99 percent, and that rarely if ever exceed 99.9 percent. Thus it is the prediction of the top 1 to 18 days of the daily census in the year that constitutes the technical challenge, and no more.

If we focus on predicting exclusively the top 5 percent, i.e., 18 days of daily census, it follows that the most important and even the only useful input data come from precisely those days. If the challenge is reformulated as one of identifying a model that accurately predicts the top 18 census levels, given the ADC, the possibility arises of adapting the normal distribution model rather than rejecting it. If the standard deviations derived from the square root of ADC estimate and a full $\sqrt{\dfrac{\Sigma\,(x - \bar{x})^2}{n - 1}}$ calculation fail to do the job, then perhaps some other method will produce a useful substitute.

In pursuit of such a substitute, an attempt was made to calculate a *synthetic* standard deviation that could be used to estimate protection levels employing the normal distribution table values (e.g., 2.33 standard deviation for 99 percent protection). This attempt involved the following steps:

- Identify the top 18 census days and ADC levels for each year's hospital census.
- Calculate the difference between each peak census day and the ADC.
- Divide each difference by the number of standard deviations each peak census day would theoretically be above the mean or ADC.
- Calculate the average of the results in step 3 for all 18 days.

For example, Table 14-10 illustrates how such a procedure was applied to a hospital with an ADC of 172.9 in 1980. The synthetic standard deviation for this hospital was 19.4. The actual standard deviation, based on all 365 days of census, was calculated as 27.0, due greatly to extremely low census days around Christmas and New Year's (lows such as 134 on Christmas Day, 140 on New Year's Day) and during the summer (129 on July 5, 130 on June 28 and July 4, 126 on August 29, for example). Such a standard deviation would have predicted a peak census day of 172.9 + 2.78(27.0) = 248 in contrast to the actual peak of 227. In contrast the square root model would have predicted the standard deviation at $\sqrt{172.9}$ = 13.15 and the peak daily census at 172.9 + 2.78(13.15) = 209. In other words the actual peak census was roughly halfway between these two other estimates and close to neither one.

A similar procedure was employed for 300 hospital-years of daily census data, with information from hospitals of varying sizes in eight states. The synthetic standard deviations derived from these measures predicted actual peak daily census levels with a mean error of only 1.37 percent.

The challenge is not to derive synthetic standard deviations and predictions of peak census levels from actual data. Because observed data are the basis for such derivations, observed data make a better basis for making bed need decisions than predictive models anyway. The challenge is to develop estimates of peak daily census levels based on ADC levels fore-

**Table 14-10** Calculation of Synthetic Standard Deviation

ADC = 172.9

| (1)<br>Peak<br>Census Rank | (2)<br><br>Observation | (3)<br>Observation<br>− ADC | (4)<br>Expected*<br>z-Value | (3) ÷ (4) |
|---|---|---|---|---|
| Highest | 227 | 54.1 | 2.78 | 19.5 |
| 2nd | 221 | 48.1 | 2.54 | 18.9 |
| 3rd | 220 | 47.1 | 2.40 | 19.6 |
| 4th | 219 | 46.1 | 2.29 | 20.1 |
| 5th | 217 | 44.1 | 2.21 | 20.0 |
| 6th | 216 | 43.1 | 2.14 | 20.1 |
| 7th | 216 | 43.1 | 2.07 | 20.8 |
| 8th | 210 | 37.1 | 2.02 | 18.4 |
| 9th | 210 | 37.1 | 1.97 | 18.8 |
| 10th | 209 | 36.1 | 1.92 | 18.8 |
| 11th | 208 | 35.1 | 1.88 | 18.7 |
| 12th | 208 | 35.1 | 1.84 | 19.1 |
| 13th | 207 | 34.1 | 1.80 | 18.9 |
| 14th | 207 | 34.1 | 1.77 | 19.3 |
| 15th | 207 | 34.1 | 1.74 | 19.6 |
| 16th | 206 | 33.1 | 1.71 | 19.4 |
| 17th | 206 | 33.1 | 1.68 | 19.7 |
| 18th | 205 | 32.1 | 1.65 | 19.5 |
| | | | Mean | 19.4 |

*Expected values are derived from normal distribution table probabilities; $1/365$ = .0027 probability, which corresponds to a table value 2.78 standard deviation above the mean, for example.

cast. By accurately predicting peak daily census levels, optimal bed capacity levels for each future year can be determined.

To address this challenge, the data from all 300 hospital cases were analyzed by comparing the synthetic standard deviation (SSD) to the ADC for each case. A log-linear regression using the expression SSD = 1.34 $ADC^{.482}$ proved to have excellent predictive value ($r^2$ = .909, $p<.001$).

Although this $r^2$ value is extraordinarily high for data derived from divergent cases, it does not truly measure the predictive value of the synthetic standard deviation. To test its predictive value, the regression-predicted SSDs were used to predict actual peak daily census levels in each of the 300 cases. The errors for predictions based on formula-predicted SSD levels were higher than from actual SSD values but were still far less than errors resulting from the square root model or actual standard deviations. Specifically the mean error for SSD predictions was 2.13 percent versus 7.7 percent for the square root model and 9.2 percent from the actual standard deviation.

The conclusion of this analysis is not that the formula SSD = 1.34 ADC$^{.482}$ be universally adopted as a replacement to existing probability models for determining bed need. For one thing, the 300 hospitals from which the expression was derived do not constitute a random statistical sample of all U.S. hospitals. For another they describe past relationships between ADC and peak daily census levels and may not apply as well in the future. Third, they describe how daily census actually does vary in hospitals rather than how it might be managed.

The ability to predict peak daily census is of significant value in hospital bed need determination. It is only one of the necessary data inputs to such a process, however. The number of beds filled on a given day does not fully describe the hospital's ability to accommodate more patients. Because of multiple-bed rooms and rules against mixing incompatible patients (smokers and nonsmokers, males and females, for example) the hospital may be effectively full even with some beds empty. On the other hand hospitals have repeatedly demonstrated that they can accommodate far more patients than their official capacity when necessary.

Moreover the number of beds filled during peak demand periods of one year is not the proper basis for determining hospital capacity when that capacity will suffice for many more than one year. The pattern of annual changes in the ADC and the peak ADC year for any proposed capacity should be estimated before proper capacity can be determined in a responsible manner. Being able to predict peak daily census levels in the peak ADC year should greatly assist in determining required capacity. Estimating peak daily census levels in other years of lower ADC should assist in staffing and other demand-related planning, at least.

The synthetic standard deviation does well, especially when compared to competing models, in performing one explicit function. Once the ADC is known, the SSD predicts the level and frequency of peak daily census levels where neither bed limitations nor admissions scheduling constrain the variability of daily census. It is likely that at least during peak ADC years the pattern of daily census variations is constrained by one or both of these factors. Where this is not true, or in off-peak years, this model should be extremely accurate and of significant practical value to planners and managers.

## SUMMARY

Variability of utilization within the year is an unfortunate reality to planners and administrators because of its impact on occupancy and efficiency and subsequently on expenditures and revenues. Such variability may arise from "natural" causes in the environment or patterns of disease or from personal preferences of patients and physicians. They may be partially controlled but cannot be totally eliminated.

Techniques for forecasting the variability of utilization range from simple ratios to statistical techniques. Part-to-whole and relative average ratios may be calculated and used to forecast day-of-the-week, hour-of-the-day, or month-of-the-year fluctuations in demand. Fluctuation patterns may be combined to forecast expected use during a given hour on a given day of a given week in a given month. Where fluctuations follow a cyclical pattern, a Fourier regression may be used to forecast use at a given point in time.

Statistical distributions may be used to forecast the extent and overall pattern of variations rather than their precise timing. Empirical analysis has shown that the Poisson and normal statistical distributions have limited applicability to fluctuations in daily hospital census, however. A slightly modified approach based on a synthetic standard deviation promises to do a superior job of forecasting the extent and frequency of peak census levels, assuming that they are the chief focus of forecasting efforts, once the annual average daily census is known.

---

### Annotated Bibliography

**Brower, F.** "Feasibility of a 5-Day Medical-Surgical Unit." *Hospital Administration Currents,* January–February 1977, p. 1.

Examines the possibility of incorporating day-of-the-week variations into operation of a hospital by closing entire units when census is low on weekends.

**Cowen, J.** "Does Poisson Approximate Census Fluctuations in Planning for Hospital Bed Need?" Paper presented at the annual meeting of the American Public Health Association, New York, November 1979.

Examines daily census fluctuations in a number of hospital units, discovering that statistical models can underestimate the extent of peak census variations.

**Drosness, D., et al.** "Uses of Daily Census Data in Determining Efficiency of Units." *Hospitals,* December 1, 1967, p. 23.

Examines patterns of daily census data as they occur in hospitals, as an important factor in limiting how efficient the hospital can be.

**DuFour, R.** "Predicting Hospital Bed Needs." *Health Services Research* 9, no. 1 (Spring 1974): 61.

Describes analysis of specific unit daily census variations, showing how the pattern can be truncated by insufficient capacity and suggesting that the Poisson estimate of the standard deviation as equal to square root of ADC may underestimate variability.

**Hancock, W., et al.** "Admission Scheduling and Control Systems." III.2 in *Cost Control in Hospitals,* edited by J. Griffith et al. Ann Arbor: Health Administration Press, 1976, p. 150.

Discusses ways to control daily census variability.

**MacStravic, R.** "Areawide Fluctuations in Hospital Daily Census." *Medical Care* 17, no. 12 (December 1979): 1229.

Describes patterns of variation in daily census within a given year across groups of hospitals rather than individual institutions.

**Roemer, M.** "Bed Supply and Hospital Utilization: A Natural Experiment." *Hospitals,* November 1, 1961, p. 36.

The origin of the Roemer effect theory, speculating that as more beds are built, they tend to be filled, hence suggesting that supplies of beds be kept to a minimum.

**Shonick, W.** "Understanding the Nature of the Random Fluctuations of the Hospital Daily Census." *Medical Care* 10, no. 2 (March–April 1972): 118.

A classic discussion of the use of statistical models to predict daily census fluctuations and the effect of any given bed supply on the ability to accommodate such fluctuations.

**Weckwerth, V.** "Determining Bed Needs from Occupancy and Census Figures." *Hospitals,* January 1, 1966, p. 52.

Discusses the use of a statistical model, the Poisson-normal distribution, to predict daily census variations and determine bed needs for any given year.

# Chapter 15

# Year-to-Year Changes in Health Services Utilization

In most cases the resources of a health services organization are largely fixed over a multiyear period. An organization's physical plant and equipment cannot be adjusted annually with changing levels of utilization. Personnel and supplies can be altered to some extent, though not always in direct proportion to the extent of changes in utilization from year to year. As long as use of health services by a population changes from year to year, and their selection of one provider versus another also changes, each provider can expect changes in its annual utilization volume.

## CAPACITY LIFETIME

Although daily and seasonal changes in utilization have been studied intensively, annual changes have largely been ignored. Hospital bed need discussions have all but invariably focused on utilization expected in a single year rather than on the volume expected throughout the period when beds would be fixed. Yet it is inescapably clear that hospital bed capacity, as any other fixed resource, must be adequate, without being excessive, for whatever period it will operate. It is not possible to fix the proper resource level for a multiyear period unless the utilization expected for that period is examined.

The period that must be examined can be thought of as a *capacity lifetime*. This is the number of years over which a resource capacity is essentially fixed. In planning resource capacity, this lifetime would begin whenever the capacity would be operative and end whenever a new capacity level would be implemented. This is not the same as the life cycle or expected life of the resource itself but merely the period over which a given resource capacity level is maintained.

For capital equipment, for example, a provider may operate with one CT scanner for 5 years, then add another. The capacity lifetime for the first one-scanner capacity would thus be 5 years, even if the scanner itself is used for 10 or even if the actual scanner is replaced within the 5-year period. For physical plant capacity a lifetime is the number of years between construction projects that alter that capacity. Given the cost of construction, the amount of time and effort required to plan and implement construction projects, and the disruption that they cause in operations, physical plant capacity lifetimes are likely to be many years in length.

The beginning of a capacity lifetime would be as many months or years into the future as needed to create that new capacity. For personnel, supplies, and equipment, that may be from days to many months or even more than a year in some cases. For physical plant it is likely to be many years. Hospitals, for example, plan on three to five years before new physical plant capacity can be developed, given the planning, regulation, financing, and other hurdles involved. In such cases the lifetime for a new physical plant capacity level would begin three to five years from the time the planning process is initiated.

The length of a capacity lifetime may be a few days or months to decades. For supplies, personnel, and equipment, wherever they can be added to or reduced in a short period, their capacity lifetimes may be quite short. For physical plant, however, minimum lifetimes are likely to be years, while maximums may reach 20, 30, or more years. A hospital might operate with the same licensed bed capacity for a half century or more, even though it replaces its physical plant. For purposes of planning, a physical plant capacity lifetime would extend to the point when the basic physical plant is replaced and the capacity level could thereby be changed.

With capacity lifetimes of as few as 5 and as many as 30 years, hospital bed capacity represents a particularly appropriate example of the importance of year-to-year changes in utilization. As true for all resources with capacity lifetimes measured in years, the significance of year-to-year changes in utilization rests with two characteristics of such changes: the basic linear trend in annual utilization and the patterns of fluctuations around that trend.

The trend portrays the typical expected pattern of annual utilization, increasing or decreasing by uniform amounts each year. The mean annual utilization in the trend would indicate the average productivity of a resource during its capacity lifetime. In a hospital this would be expressed in terms of an average occupancy. If the annual average daily census of a hospital trends from 100 to 120 over a capacity lifetime, its expected mean ADC would be $(100 + 120) \div 2 = 110$ based on a linear trend. If it operated

150 beds over that lifetime, its average lifetime occupancy would be 110 ÷ 150 = 73.3%.

## FLUCTUATIONS

The fluctuations around the trend would partly determine whether the lifetime capacity level is adequate. If annual ADC levels varied as much as plus or minus 10 around the underlying trend, then an ADC as high as 120 + 10 = 130 might occur. With 150 beds it might be difficult, even impossible, to accommodate the daily fluctuations in demand expected around an ADC of 130. Based on previous discussions (Chapter 14) the expected synthetic standard deviation for an ADC of 130 would be $1.34(130^{.482}) = 14.0$. With 150 beds available there would be only 150 − 130 = 20 beds or 20 ÷ 14.0 = 1.429 standard deviations of reserve capacity available. All 150 beds would be expected to be full 28 days of the year. With problems mixing incompatible patients in multibed rooms, the 150-bed capacity might be effectively full 50 or 60 days of the year.

In order to determine whether a proposed capacity is likely to be adequate for a given capacity lifetime or to decide when to modify a resource's capacity, both the trend and expected fluctuation pattern of utilization must be considered. The trend determines how long a capacity lifetime can be, which in turn influences the likely pattern of annual fluctuations. The pattern of fluctuations in annual utilization determines whether a capacity level proposed for or operated during a lifetime period is adequate.

### Factors

The reasons for year-to-year fluctuations in annual ADC levels are many and varied. Principal among them are demographic, health system, and psychographic factors. In theory a careful analysis might be aimed at predicting the precise pattern expected in a given hospital case. In practice, however, the factors are likely to work in complex and unpredictable ways. Because the pattern of year-to-year fluctuations is predictable on a random statistical basis, this is likely to be sufficient for most decisions.

Demographic factors that can produce variations as well as trends in use of health services primarily relate to health status. Occasional flu epidemics, for example, can drive up utilization in one year, while the absence of an epidemic can hold down utilization in another. Changes in attitudes toward family size or in employment levels can produce variations in obstetric and total utilization. Any factor that significantly influences utilization and that fluctuates significantly from year to year can produce fluctuations in utilization.

Health system factors include changes in provider numbers or types and changes in health insurance. In a small hospital the addition or departure of one physician can create significant fluctuations. Even in larger hospitals a major influx or outflux of physicians can produce significant variations in the numbers and types of patients admitted. A nurses' strike can force utilization down in one hospital and up in others. The size of the hospital can greatly inhibit year-to-year variability if occupancy is high. The lack of beds to enable census to go any higher may produce steady, high occupancy in a particular hospital, meaning that patients are going elsewhere in peak demand years.

Psychographic factors in both physicians and patients can also be influential. A malpractice scandal, an effective marketing program, and changes in ownership or administration can greatly affect the relative preference for one hospital over another. Such shifts are hard to predict in the long run, and subject to deliberate strategic efforts as well, hence difficult to incorporate in an effort at forecasting a long-term pattern of fluctuation.

**Trends**

A trend in annual utilization can be of any slope in practice, upward or downward, gradual, steep, or even flat. Its slope determines how long a given capacity is adequate. With a model of daily census variation within a year, it is possible to determine a maximum ADC level that can be acceptably accommodated in any capacity. A forecast trend in annual utilization would then indicate when that maximum ADC is expected to occur or be exceeded.

For example, a 150-bed capacity might have its maximum acceptable ADC calculated as follows:

- Maximum turnaway is set at 2½ percent of the time, i.e., 9 days per year.
- Reserve capacity required for 97½ percent protection; i.e., 2½ percent turnaway, is 1.96 standard deviations.
- ADC level is as close as possible to but not less than 1.96 of its standard deviation below 150.
- Answer is calculated by trial and error; 123.2 ADC has a standard deviation of $1.34(123.2^{.482}) = 13.64$; $1.96 \times 13.64 = 26.73$; $123.2 + 26.73 = 149.93$. Hence 123.2 is highest ADC that can be accommo-

dated in 150 beds with 97½ percent protection or 2½ percent turnaway.

If the first year in the 150-bed capacity were forecast at an ADC of 105
with an expected increase of 4.5 per year, the capacity lifetime would be
only 5 years. If the increase were 2.25 per year, the lifetime would be 9
years. If each year's ADC were only 1.0 higher than the previous year,
then the capacity lifetime would be 19 years. (See Table 15-1.) In all cases
123.0 would be the highest actual ADC because the expected ADC in the
following year would be greater than the maximum ADC of 123.2.

The mean ADC level in all three cases would be the same, (105 + 123)
÷ 2 = 114.0. In a linear trend the mean ADC is a function of the low and
high ADC levels and independent of the length of the capacity lifetime.
Whether the 150-bed capacity would truly suffice for a given lifetime,
however, is a function of the variability in ADC levels around the underlying trend, as well as the trend itself. Variability is partly a function of
the length of the capacity lifetime.

**Expected Patterns**

Based on analysis of hundreds of cases, involving both individual hospitals and whole systems of facilities, the pattern of fluctuations in annual

**Table 15-1** Capacity Lifetime

| 5 Years | 9 Years | 19 Years |
|---|---|---|
| 105.0 | 105.0 | 105.0 |
| 109.5 | 107.25 | 106.0 |
| 114.0 | 109.5 | 107.0 |
| 118.5 | 111.75 | 108.0 |
| 123.0 | 114.0 | 109.0 |
| | 116.25 | 110.0 |
| | 118.5 | 111.0 |
| | 120.75 | 112.0 |
| | 123.0 | 113.0 |
| | | 114.0 |
| | | 115.0 |
| | | 116.0 |
| | | 117.0 |
| | | 118.0 |
| | | 119.0 |
| | | 120.0 |
| | | 121.0 |
| | | 122.0 |
| | | 123.0 |

ADC levels around their multiyear trend tends to follow a pattern based on the normal statistical distribution. This pattern represents the expected distribution of individual observations in a small random sample, expressed in terms of the sample's mean and standard error (s.e.). The extent and overall pattern of fluctuations are a function of the number of observations in the sample, hence the number of years in a capacity lifetime.

The expected patterns of variability for samples of 5, 9, and 19 observations are shown in Table 15-2. The pattern demonstrates perfect symmetry with fluctuations below the mean (minus) exactly duplicating those above the mean (plus). It also shows a greater extent of fluctuation with larger numbers of observations. Thus, in a 5-year lifetime the maximum expected fluctuation above the trend would be plus or minus 1.163 standard errors. For a 9-year lifetime the maximum deviation would be plus or minus 1.485 standard errors, while in a 19-year lifetime it would be plus or minus 1.844 standard errors. The key is to estimate the standard error in each case.

No theoretical model predicts the standard error of annual ADC levels around their trend. Based on analysis of actual experience in hundreds of cases, the standard error of annual ADC levels in individual hospitals has averaged .527 MADC$^{.545}$ ($r^2 = .845$, $p<.001$) where MADC is the mean average daily census for the multiyear capacity lifetime. With a mean ADC of 114.0 the standard error of individual annual ADC levels would be .527(114.0$^{.545}$) = 6.93.

---

**Table 15-2** Variability Patterns

| 5 Observations | 9 Observations | 19 Observations |
|---|---|---|
| − 1.163 se | − 1.485 se | − 1.844 se |
| − 0.495 se | − 0.932 se | − 1.380 se |
| mean | − 0.572 se | − 1.099 se |
| + 0.495 se | − 0.275 se | − 0.886 se |
| + 1.163 se | mean | − 0.707 se |
| | + 0.275 se | − 0.548 se |
| | + 0.572 se | − 0.402 se |
| | + 0.932 se | − 0.264 se |
| | + 1.485 se | − 0.131 se |
| | | mean |
| | | + 0.131 se |
| | | + 0.264 se |
| | | + 0.402 se |
| | | + 0.548 se |
| | | + 0.707 se |
| | | etc. |

Over a 5-year lifetime the maximum expected deviation around the trend would be plus or minus 1.163 standard errors, or 1.163(6.93) = 8.06. Thus the range of fluctuation would be plus or minus 8.06 around the trend. In a 9-year lifetime, it would be ± (1.485)(6.93) = 10.29. In 19 years it would be ± (1.844)(6.93) = 12.78. The problem is, When will the maximum deviation around the trend occur? If it happens during the first year of the forecast trend, it could produce an ADC as high as 105.0 + 8.06 = 113.06 in a 5-year lifetime, 105.0 + 10.24 = 115.24 in a 9-year period, or 105.0 + 12.78 = 117.78 in a 19-year period. All such ADC levels could be accommodated in the 150-bed capacity because it is adequate up to an ADC of 123.0.

If maximum deviation occurs at the end of the forecast trend, it could produce an expected high of 123.0 + 8.06 = 131.06 in 5 years, 123.0 + 10.24 = 133.24 in 9 years, or 123.0 + 12.78 = 135.78 in 19 years. The 150-bed capacity would be inadequate in all three situations with a maximum intended ADC of 123.0. If maximum deviation occurs toward the end rather than the beginning of an upward trend, the capacity may be inadequate or the lifetime too long, depending on one's perspective.

In the absence of any reason for expecting maximum fluctuation to occur early versus late in the lifetime trend, the only unbiased estimate is that it will occur at the midpoint of the trend. Thus the maximum expected ADC based on the pattern of variability would be the mean ADC plus the maximum expected deviation. In a 5-year period this would be 114.0 + 8.06 = 122.06. In a 9-year period the highest expected ADC would be 114.0 + 10.24 = 124.24. In a 19-year lifetime it would be 114.0 + 12.78 = 126.78.

Thus in both a 9-year and 19-year planned lifetime the expected pattern of fluctuations in ADC levels above the trend would produce ADC levels higher than should be accommodated by the planned capacity of 150 beds. At this point the hospital could choose to gamble that fluctuations in the future won't be what they have been but that annual ADC levels will stay closer to the trend. It could also gamble that fluctuations above the mean will tend to occur early in the capacity's lifetime. Either way the hospital could stay with the 150-bed capacity decision, as long as it is confident that the ADC will not rise above 123.0 due to random fluctuations.

If unwilling to gamble, the hospital could build a capacity adequate to the maximum expected ADC whether expected from trend or fluctuation. For a 9-year lifetime this would mean building enough capacity to handle an ADC of 124.24. Based on previous analysis of daily census variations, and holding to a 97½ percent protection standard, this would require 124.24 + (1.96)(1.34 × 124.24$^{.482}$) = 151.1, or 152 beds instead of 150. For the

19-year lifetime this would mean $126.78 + (1.96)(1.34 \times 126.78^{.482}) = 153.9$, or 154 beds.

Given that average ADC levels for the capacity lifetimes illustrated would be 114.0, the addition of beds would reduce the average lifetime occupancy achieved. With 150 beds the average lifetime occupancy would be $114 \div 150 = 76.0\%$. With 152 beds average occupancy would drop to $114 \div 152 = 75.0\%$. With 154 beds it would be only 74.0%. The hospital might prefer to gamble on fluctuations if it could not live with the lower average occupancy.

In individual cases a hospital's own past fluctuations in ADC levels might be a better basis for estimating future fluctuations than the .527 $MADC^{.545}$ formula cited. To calculate the standard error around a trend, the following process can be followed:

- Calculate the linear regression trend for past utilization (see Chapter 4).
- Take the standard deviation of the ADC levels and square it to determine the variance.
- Take the $r^2$ value for the regression and subtract it from 1.000.
- Multiply $(1 - r^2)$ times the variance.
- The square root of this unexplained variance is the standard error around the trend.

For example, with this process and yearly ADC levels of

94.3
92.1
96.4
98.6
102.0
107.7
109.3
112.0
114.7
123.8
128.6
140.2
146.1
149.1
151.6
150.5

calculations would be

$r = .9797$

$r^2 = .9598$

standard deviation $= 21.738$

standard deviation squared $= 472.56$

$1 - r^2 = .0402$

$(.0402)(472.56) = 18.997$

$\sqrt{18.997} = 4.36 =$ standard error of ADC levels around their linear trend

If utilization over time is not expected to follow any particular trend or will follow a trend with little slope, the length of a capacity lifetime can be as long as 20 or 30 years. In such cases the trend may have little impact on the lifetime capacity required, although fluctuations around the trend may determine requirements. In such cases capacity may be determined on the basis of risk or on the expected highest ADC levels over a specific lifetime.

## RISK APPROACH

If the ADC trend forecast for a planned capacity has no slope, the capacity is expected to serve the same ADC each year. Even with no slope, however, there is the expected fluctuation in ADC with which to deal. For a capacity lifetime with a mean ADC of 150, for example, the expected standard error of the ADC would be $.527(150^{.545}) = 8.05$. The probability of ADC levels of any particular value or higher can be estimated based on the normal distribution. An ADC of 2.33 standard errors above the mean should occur only 1 percent of the time, for example. One of 1.645 standard errors above the mean would be expected only 5 percent of the time.

With a long lifetime of 20 or 30 years the probability that any one of those years would have an ADC equal to or greater than a given number of standard errors above the mean ADC would be 20 or 30 times the specific probability. Thus, with an expectation of an ADC as high as 1.645 above the expected value of 5 percent, the probability of such an ADC level occurring in 20 years would be $1 - .95^{20}$, or .642. The probability of such a level occurring sometime in a 30-year cycle is $1 - .95^{30}$, or .785. Although the probability won't quite reach certainty, i.e., 1.000, probabilities this high mean that it would be quite a gamble not to have capacity sufficient for such an ADC.

If it were decided that the greatest acceptable risk would be 5 percent in 20 years, the bed capacity equal to this protection could be determined as follows: $1 - x^{20} = .050$, $x^{20} = .950$; $x = \sqrt[20]{.950} = .997$; the normal distribution table shows that a .997 one-tailed probability occurs at 2.75 standard errors above the mean. Thus a capacity equal to 2.75 standard errors above the mean would offer 95 percent assurance that its maximum acceptable ADC would not be exceeded over a 20-year period.

## EXPECTED VALUE APPROACH

Instead of choosing some arbitrary protection level, capacity over a long-term, no-trend lifetime could be determined on the basis of the expected peak ADC. In a 20-year period, for example, the peak ADC, according to order statistics, should be 1.867 standard errors above the mean ADC. If the mean ADC were 150 and the year-to-year standard error equal to $.527(150^{.545}) = 8.05$, then an ADC equal to $150 + (1.867)(8.05) = 165.0$ would be the expected peak. In order to manage 95% protection during the peak ADC year, a total of $165.0 + (1.645)(1.34 \times 165^{.482}) = 190.8$ beds would be required. If the capacity were set at 191 beds, slightly greater than 95% protection, the lifetime average occupancy would be $150 \div 191 = 78.5\%$.

Given the great uncertainty that attends forecasting, especially long-range forecasts of utilization, one possible response is to estimate the likelihood of a good or bad outcome rather than utilization itself. For example, a hospital might plan a 50-bed addition to its present 200-bed capacity. It can then determine the highest ADC level it is willing to accommodate in 250 beds. If that ADC is 225, for example, it might estimate how probable it is that its ADC level will exceed 225 before five years of whatever capacity lifetime it deems minimally acceptable.

By the same token, if it decides that it must achieve at least an 80 percent average lifetime occupancy for the new 250-bed capacity, it can estimate the likelihood that ADC levels will rise high enough to create such an average within 20 or 30 years. If it confidently expects its first-year ADC to be 180, knowing it needs an average ADC of 200 to hit 80 percent average occupancy, it need only determine how confident it can be that ADC will eventually hit 220 (assuming linear growth). Only if it is confident that such an ADC will be reached during the lifetime of the proposed capacity will it approve adding 50 beds. (See Chapter 17 for further discussion.)

## DECLINING TREND

In some past circumstances, and perhaps more future situations, annual ADC levels follow a declining trend. In such cases the pattern of variation would be expected to be the same as in an increasing trend. The decisions would be somewhat different, however, in that lead time and duration would be different. Closing a wing of the hospital, for example, in response to declining ADC might be accomplished in a matter of days or weeks rather than three to five years. A reopening of the closed wing or closure of another portion of the facility might also be accomplished on relatively short notice because no construction is involved.

In effect decisions in response to a declining utilization trend can be made reactively although those in an increasing trend should be made proactively. Moreover it is likely that the hospital will try to maintain higher protection levels in a declining census situation than in a case of planning new construction. With the physical plant already there, deliberately operating at low protection would likely cause medical staff and community outcries. Moreover the increments by which capacity would be reduced would be dictated by its *existing* physical plant configuration: the size of its nursing units, floors, or wings.

For example, a 150-bed facility might anticipate future utilization declining from a peak ADC of 123. If it intended to close a 30-bed unit, it would plan to do so at a point when expected utilization could be accommodated confortably in a $150 - 30 = 120$-bed facility. Rather than live with 97½ percent protection, however, it might not actually reduce capacity until it could expect 99 percent protection in the smaller capacity.

By trial and error it can be determined that an ADC of 92.3 is the highest that can be accommodated in a 120-bed capacity with at least 99% protection. This ADC has an expected standard deviation of 11.87. Add to this ADC a reserve capacity equal to 2.33 of its standard deviations and capacity requirements amount to 120 beds:

$$(1.34 \times 92.3^{.482}) = 11.87$$
$$2.33 \times 11.87 = 27.66$$
$$92.3 + 27.66 = 119.96 \text{ beds}$$

Thus the hospital would probably not reduce its capacity until the year in which it expected or actually experienced an ADC of 92.3 or lower. Over the capacity lifetime of the 150-bed facility the average lifetime occupancy would then be only $(92.3 + 123) \div 2 = 107.65 \div 150 = 71.8\%$. If there were significant financial or other incentives, the hospital might reduce its capacity sooner and achieve a higher average occupancy. On the other hand the decline might begin at an ADC level lower than 123 and result in an even lower lifetime average occupancy.

## CAPACITY INCREMENT

A decision to expand a hospital's capacity in anticipation of increasing utilization should obviously be made three to five years in advance of achieving the maximum acceptable ADC level in its current capacity. Deciding on how large an increment by which to expand that capacity would then be based on three considerations. First, how long a capacity lifetime would be expected in the new capacity before its maximum ADC is reached? Second, what average occupancy would be maintained during the new capacity lifetime? Third, what increment makes construction and staffing sense relative to current facilities and staffing patterns?

The length of a capacity lifetime, as discussed, should probably be at least five years in most cases. With any given trend of increasing utilization, there are likely to be a number of hypothetical options as to how large an expansion to plan. The greater the increment in added capacity, all other things being equal, the longer the lifetime for the new capacity.

The longer the lifetime and greater the increment added, however, the lower the average occupancy would be. In a case of a hospital whose maximum ADC in its present capacity is 123 for 150 beds, with expected annual increases of 4.6 per year, two options might be considered.

1. A 10-year lifetime would mean that by the tenth year the expected ADC would be $123 + (10 \times 4.6) = 169$. In order to offer $97\frac{1}{2}\%$ protection in the new capacity for 10 years, a capacity of $169 + 1.96(1.34 \times 169^{.482}) = 201$ beds would be needed, an addition of 51 beds. Over the 10 years a mean ADC of $(127.6 + 169) \div 2 = 148.3$ would be expected. (Because the ADC in the old capacity's last year was 123, the first year in the new capacity would be $123 + 4.6 = 127.6$.) With a mean ADC of 148.3 and 201 beds the average lifetime occupancy would be $148.3 \div 201 = 73.8\%$.

2. A 5-year lifetime would anticipate a peak ADC of only $123 + (5 \times 4.6) = 146$. To ensure $97\frac{1}{2}\%$ protection during the peak ADC year, a total of $146 + 1.96(1.34 \times 146^{.482}) = 176$ beds would be needed. The mean ADC during the 5-year lifetime would be $(127.6 + 146) \div 2 = 136.8$. With 176 beds the average lifetime occupancy would be $136.8 \div 176 = 77.7\%$. Over a second 5-year lifetime, with tenth-year ADC of 169, a capacity of 201 beds would be used for a mean ADC of $(150.6 + 169) \div 2 = 159.8$. The average lifetime occupancy for

the second 5 years would then be 159.8 ÷ 201 = 79.5%. For the entire 10-year period the average occupancy would be (77.7 + 79.5) ÷ 2 = 78.6% rather than the 73.8% achieved through adding one large increment.

The logic of construction and staffing represents a separate concern, not related to year-to-year fluctuations or length of capacity lifetimes. If the hospital's architecture dictates 50 beds to a floor or 30 beds to a nursing unit, the increment chosen is likely to reflect this rather than be dictated entirely by protection levels and occupancy considerations. If financing is available only for a certain amount, the size of the incremental addition might be limited by financial considerations.

The expected trend and annual fluctuation pattern of future utilization levels should provide a technical data base for making capacity decisions. It is not the sole basis for making such decisions, however. Like all decisions, selecting a new capacity should be based on all its expected consequences or all the organization's success criteria, to the extent that such can be anticipated. Adding in the inescapable realities of trends and fluctuations in ADC levels over time further complicates an already complex decision but should significantly improve the quality of the decision and its consequences.

## SUMMARY

Year-to-year changes in health services utilization have been largely forgotten, though they are a significant factor in planning and managing health services delivery programs. Hospital bed capacity, and any capital capacity with a lifetime more than one year not subject to simple annual adjustments, must serve a number of annual utilization levels. Although annual use of health services is likely to follow a trend influenced by population growth, aging, and other factors, it also fluctuates around that trend in a relatively random fashion.

The order statistics model provides a basis for predicting the extent of variability in annual hospital ADC levels around their multiyear trends. Based on empirical analysis of past annual utilization in hospitals, this model does well in predicting annual variations once the standard error of the long-term trend is known. This same analysis suggests that the standard error can be fairly accurately predicted as a function of the long-term mean ADC level in each case.

Once the pattern of long-term annual utilization levels is forecast, more reasonable decisions regarding the timing and size of capacity adjustments can be made. In order to do so, specific choices must be made regarding the maximum acceptable one-year occupancy, minimum acceptable average occupancy, and optimum increment for capacity adjustments. These in turn require explicit anticipation of and trade-offs among the performance consequences of utilization levels in the context of whatever capacity is available.

### Annotated Bibliography

Dixon, W. and Massey, F. *Introduction to Statistical Analysis*. New York: McGraw-Hill, 1969, pp. 133–134.

Discusses order statistics; the table on p. 489 presents expected dispersion of observations in samples up to 20.

MacStravic, R. "Average Life Cycle Occupancy: A Radical New Approach to Bed Needs and Appropriateness Review Decisions." *Health Care Planning and Marketing* 1, no. 1 (April 1981): 25; "Admissions Scheduling and Capacity Pooling: Minimizing Hospital Bed Requirements." *Inquiry* 18, no. 4 (Winter 1981): 345.

These latter two articles are the only discussions available in the literature on the importance of year-to-year changes in hospital utilization for planning and operation of hospitals.

# Chapter 16

# A Forecast Early Warning System

In Chapters 14 and 15 the focus was on predicting patterns of variation in short periods based on a forecast of utilization covering a longer period. If patterns of variation in utilization are both consistent and persistent, they can also be used to do the opposite. This chapter examines a technique for predicting utilization covering a long period based on observed utilization during a shorter period. This technique offers a way of developing early warnings that prior forecasts might have been in error.

The data base and analysis required are the same as that used in predicting the expected utilization within one period based on the pattern of fluctuating utilization observed over larger periods. To illustrate with a simple example, consider the relationship between days of the week and the full week's utilization. Table 16-1 uses the same ratios as in previous chapters.

If Monday's utilization happens to be 48 visits, the full week is estimated at 48 ÷ .16 = 300 visits. If Tuesday's utilization is 52 visits, the combination of Monday and Tuesday would produce the expectation that the week will have (48 + 52) ÷ (.16 + .14), or 100 ÷ .30 = 333 visits. Similar calculations can be made with each additional day.

## PRECISION AND ACCURACY

In general we would expect the precision of each early warning estimate to increase as each additional day is included. Because one day represents only a small portion of the whole week, it is likely that its relationship to the entire week's utilization varied substantially in the past. This would be reflected in the standard deviation of past ratios. The ratio of Monday's utilization to the whole week has a mean value of .16 in this example, with a standard deviation of .03. In other words only about two-thirds of the time were past ratios within the range of .16 plus or minus .03 or between .13 and .19. With 48 visits on Monday we can have only 68 percent confidence that the week's utilization will be between 48 ÷ .19 = 253 and 48 ÷ .13 = 369. To be 95 percent sure, we'd have to use a range of plus or minus 1.96 standard deviations, or roughly between ratios of .10 and .22. This would give us a potential range of 48 ÷ .22 = 218 up to 48 ÷ .10 = 480.

Such extreme ranges are likely to be all but useless as warning devices. There would be little comfort in an estimate that utilization for the week is almost surely (95 percent confidence) 218 to 480 visits. None of the individual days promise much better precision, though Tuesday shows a 95 percent confidence interval smaller than any other day at .14 plus or minus 1.96(.02) or roughly .10 to .18. By adding the days together, however, we would expect precision to increase dramatically.

For example, Monday and Tuesday together represent .16 plus .14, or .30, of the week's utilization. With only four of six days left, the combination of the two days is likely to yield a more precise and reliable estimate of the week's utilization than would only one day. Adding a third day and a fourth would increase precision and reliability even more, though decreasing the early aspect of the early warning. The data in Table 16-2

**Table 16-1** Days of the Week and Utilization

| Day | Mean Ratio | Standard Deviation |
|---|---|---|
| Monday | .16 | .03 |
| Tuesday | .14 | .02 |
| Wednesday | .18 | .03 |
| Thursday | .17 | .03 |
| Friday | .20 | .04 |
| Saturday | .15 | .03 |

**Table 16-2** Sets of Days and Standard Deviation

| Days | Mean Ratio | Standard Deviation |
|---|---|---|
| Monday | .16 | .030 |
| MT | .30 | .020 |
| MTW | .48 | .015 |
| MTWT | .65 | .010 |
| MTWTF | .85 | .005 |
| MTWTFS | 1.00 | .000 |

might describe the precision of sets of days taken together in predicting a full week's utilization.

Thus, the combination of Monday and Tuesday has a standard deviation of .20. Although this is the same value as for Tuesday alone, it produces greater precision because it applies to a larger mean ratio value. A 95 percent confidence interval for Monday and Tuesday's ratio of .30 would be roughly .26 to .34. With 100 visits for the two days the estimate for the week would be total visits between $100 \div .34 = 294$ and $100 \div 26 = 385$. The estimate based on Tuesday alone would have a confidence interval between .10 and .18 applied to 52 visits. Its prediction would be the week's visits between $52 \div .18 = 288$ and $52 \div .10 = 520$, a much larger range.

Adding in Wednesday's visits would increase precision. If there were 50 more visits on Wednesday, giving a total of 150 so far for the week, the mean ratio estimate for the week would be $150 \div .48 = 313$ visits. With a standard deviation of .015 the 95 percent confidence interval for the ratio would be roughly .48 plus or minus .03, or between .45 and .51. The resulting prediction would be between $150 \div .51 = 294$ and $150 \div .45 = 333$, a much more reasonable range.

Employing this technique in practice provides a classic example of information trade-off in decision making. The earlier the information is, hence the more useful for making decisions, the more imprecise it is, hence the greater the uncertainty in making a decision. The later the information is, the greater the precision, hence confidence in the decision, but the less time there is for the decision to be effective. By Thursday, for example, it may be too late to increase or decrease staff in response to a high or low forecast. Moreover there would be only three days left for the consequences of a decision to be felt. If expenses must be cut in anticipation of lower revenue, for example, they must be cut twice as much if applied to only three days as if applied to six.

## EARLIER WARNINGS

Because there is such value in getting as early a warning as possible and because utilization tends to be fairly stable or at least highly autocorrelated over time in most cases, there exists the possibility of developing even earlier warnings via the same technique. Using the days of the week example, we might try to obtain early estimates of one week's utilization by examining the utilization of the last few days of the prior week. If there is a consistent and persistent relationship between the number of visits on Friday and Saturday of one week and the total number of visits during the following week, an even more useful early warning might be obtained.

The days of the prior week could also be added to the early days of this week to yield more precise estimates.

To secure the necessary ratios and standard deviations, data on past weeks would be analyzed. The number of visits on Friday of one week would be divided by the total visits of the following week in each case. At least 10 such pairs should be analyzed for an adequate picture of the relationship. As true with the within-the-week ratios, there is a choice as to which weeks to use. If there tends to be a different day of the week pattern in different times of the year, it would be best to look at the same week in previous years to obtain mean ratios and standard deviations. If no such seasonal variability exists, and the pattern has changed over time, the most recent weeks would be preferred. As true for all prediction techniques, a subjective judgment is required in selecting the number and set of time periods to be used in calculating past relationships, as well as in the choice of relying on such relationships to forecast the future.

The data in Table 16-3 represent a possible set of mean ratios and standard deviations based on prior days' utilization in combination with days early in the week of interest.

With this information a forecast of next week's utilization can be developed with data from this week. If Friday of this week has 60 visits, for example, the early warning estimate for next week would be $60 \div .19 = 316$ visits. The 95 percent confidence range would be based on ratios roughly between .11 and .27 or from $60 \div .27 = 222$ and $60 \div .11 = 545$.

A more precise estimate could be derived by combining Friday and Saturday visit volumes. If Saturday has 50 visits, for example, the early warning estimate for next week would be $50 + 60 = 110 \div .33 = 333$ visits. The confidence range in this case would be roughly .25 to .41 for a prediction range of $110 \div .41 = 268$ to $110 \div .25 = 440$.

If this is not precise enough to act on, the actual visits on Monday can be added to increase precision and reliability. If Monday's visits amount to 60, for example, the combined total of $110 + 60 = 170$ visits would produce an early warning prediction of $170 \div .49 = 347$ visits for the

**Table 16-3** Mean Ratios and Standard Deviations

| Days | Mean Ratio | Standard Deviation |
|------|------------|--------------------|
| Friday | .19 | .04 |
| FS | .33 | .04 |
| FSM | .49 | .03 |
| FSMT | .63 | .02 |
| FSMTW | .80 | .01 |

week. The 95 percent confidence range would be roughly between ratios of .43 and .55, so the prediction for the week would be between 170 ÷ .55 = 309 and 170 ÷ .43 = 395.

With Tuesday's volume added, even further precision is possible. If there are 50 visits on Tuesday, or a total of 220 for the four days, the early warning forecast would be 220 ÷ .63 = 349 visits for the week. The confidence range of the ratios would be roughly .59 to .67, so the forecast range would be from 220 ÷ .67 = 328 to 220 ÷ .59 = 373. At some point, precision is likely to be good enough to make a confident decision and early enough to be effective.

## ACTUAL APPLICATION

The previous example of day-of-the-week variations is for illustration only. In a given situation ratios may or may not be consistent enough in the past to enable precise enough forecasts early enough to make decisions. Even where past relationships are consistent, there may be concern over their persistence, though only immediate-term persistence is required. To provide an example of an actual application, the following case of hospital fiscal year utilization is offered.

Four hospitals in a multihospital system operate on fiscal years beginning on July 1. They submit budgets based on their next-year utilization forecasts in March. Such forecasts are based on utilization in previous years and the first nine months of the present fiscal year, adjusted for estimated changes in the dynamics of their local situation and their expected effects. The financial target of such budgets is the difference between revenues and expenditures, the bottom line needed to meet capital requirements for each hospital.

If utilization looks as if it will be significantly below budget, and action can be taken early enough, the hospitals can choose among the following strategies:

- consciously seeking to increase utilization, through physician recruitment, for example
- increasing charges so as to augment revenues even with lower volume
- decreasing expenditures via personnel cuts or other reductions

The earlier such actions can be taken, the longer each can be effective. The longer the potential effect, the less dramatic the action need be because it can be multiplied by many months of experience. If action is taken late, however, and few months are left to overcome significant discrepancies between budgeted revenues and expenditures, the action would have to be fairly drastic. There might not be enough time to implement an effective marketing strategy. If charges are to be increased, they probably must be increased dramatically because few patient days are left to recover lost revenue. If expenses are to be cut, large numbers of employees might have to be laid off, for example.

The following ratios and standard deviations were derived from examining the most recent 10 years of utilization experience in each hospital. Care had to be taken in analyzing such data, however. In one hospital the most recent 3 years' experiences were not included in analysis. In each of those 3 years nurses' strikes during the summer significantly distorted the relationships between summer months' utilization and that for the year as a whole. In another hospital changes in the medical staff specialty mix and services had altered the pattern of seasonal variation, so only the most recent 6 years' data were used.

The ratios in Tables 16-4 through 16-7 reflect the results of the analysis. The first set of ratios cover the three months before the new fiscal year. The second set indicates ratios for these prior year months in conjunction with the early months of the new fiscal year. The third set covers ratios for months in the new fiscal year only. The fourth column in the tables is the *estimated* confidence interval for each ratio, based on plus or minus 1.96 standard deviations divided by the mean. The actual confidence interval is close to the estimate, though being based on division by ratios is not symmetrical.

A confidence interval of plus or minus .05 around a ratio of .20, for example, would have a range below the mean forecast of 20 percent of the forecast value. The range above the forecast would be 33⅓ percent, however. Dividing by .20 is the same as multiplying by 5. Dividing by .25 equals multiplying by 4. Dividing by .15 equals multiplying by 6⅔. Thus, the estimated range would be plus or minus .05 divided by .20, or plus or minus 25 percent, while the actual range would be from minus 20 percent to plus 33⅓ percent. The estimate provides at least a general picture of the confidence range, though the actual range of forecasts is always asymmetrical, with greater range above than below the mean ratio forecast.

The tables illustrate some expected realities related to seasonal patterns of variations in utilization. First of all, each hospital's pattern tends to differ from the others. The hospital in Table 16-4, for example, has a much higher proportion of its annual utilization during the summer months compared to the other three. July represents 8.5 percent of the year's total with July–August combined representing 17.68 percent. This is quite a bit larger than the proportion expected based on the number of days in these two months (62 divided by 365 equals 16.9 percent). In contrast the other

**Table 16-4** 45-Bed Hospital

| Period | Mean Ratio | Standard Deviation | Estimated Confidence Interval |
|---|---|---|---|
| April | .0817 | .0069 | ± 16.6% |
| May | .0871 | .0096 | ± 21.6% |
| June | .0804 | .0095 | ± 23.2% |
| AM | .1688 | .0174 | ± 20.2% |
| MJ | .1675 | .0159 | ± 18.6% |
| AMJ | .2518 | .0217 | ± 16.9% |
| JJ | .1654 | .0182 | ± 21.6% |
| JJA | .2572 | .0174 | ± 13.3% |
| JJAS | .3486 | .0185 | ± 10.4% |
| MJJ | .2525 | .0252 | ± 19.7% |
| MJJA | .3443 | .0207 | ± 11.6% |
| MJJAS | .4357 | .0306 | ± 14.0% |
| AMJJ | .3342 | .0292 | ± 17.1% |
| AMJJA | .4264 | .0222 | ± 10.2% |
| AMJJAS | .5178 | .0247 | ± 9.3% |
| July | .0850 | .0102 | ± 23.5% |
| JA | .1768 | .0080 | ± 8.8% |
| JAS | .2682 | .0083 | ± 6.1% |
| JASO | .3586 | .0131 | ± 7.2% |
| JASON | .4380 | .0092 | ± 4.1% |
| JASOND | .5076 | .0076 | ± 2.9% |
| JASONDJ | .5938 | .0130 | ± 4.3% |
| JASONDJF | .6624 | .0160 | ± 4.7% |
| JASONDJFM | .7424 | .0270 | ± 7.1% |

hospitals experience only 14.61 percent to 16.01 percent of their annual utilization during these two months. Each hospital's ratios are likely to be idiosyncratic to its situation.

Another indication in these tables is an expected suggestion that the *extent* of variability from month to month is greater in smaller hospitals than in larger. As illustrated in Chapter 14 daily census variability is *relatively* greater for smaller ADC levels. Thus the range of monthly ratios in the small hospital is far greater than in the large. The ratio for February is only .0686, for example (July–February's .6624 minus July–January's .5938 equals .0686) while that for August is .0918 (July–August's .1768 minus July's .0850 equals .0918). The range for the large hospital is only from September's .0791 to January's .0888, less than half the range of the small hospital.

A third finding is that the variability in monthly ratios from *year to year* is far greater in the small hospital than in the large. This is illustrated by

**Table 16-5** 105-Bed Hospital

| Period | Mean Ratio | Standard Deviation | Estimated Confidence Interval |
|---|---|---|---|
| April | .0833 | .0041 | ± 9.6% |
| May | .0851 | .0060 | ± 13.8% |
| June | .0810 | .0061 | ± 14.8% |
| AM | .1684 | .0087 | ± 10.1% |
| MJ | .1661 | .0094 | ± 10.3% |
| AMJ | .2494 | .0118 | ± 10.1% |
| JJ | .1543 | .0104 | ± 13.3% |
| JJA | .2271 | .0084 | ± 7.3% |
| JJAS | .3058 | .0098 | ± 6.4% |
| MJJ | .2394 | .0111 | ± 9.1% |
| MJJA | .3122 | .0099 | ± 6.2% |
| MJJAS | .3909 | .0112 | ± 5.6% |
| AMJJ | .3227 | .0125 | ± 7.6% |
| AMJJA | .3955 | .0111 | ± 5.5% |
| AMJJAS | .4742 | .0116 | ± 4.8% |
| July | .0733 | .0056 | ± 15.0% |
| JA | .1461 | .0063 | ± 8.5% |
| JAS | .2248 | .0038 | ± 3.3% |
| JASO | .3123 | .0080 | ± 5.0% |
| JASON | .3960 | .0119 | ± 5.9% |
| JASOND | .4754 | .0056 | ± 2.3% |
| JASONDJ | .5617 | .0060 | ± 2.1% |
| JASONDJF | .6411 | .0065 | ± 2.0% |
| JASONDJFM | .7344 | .0067 | ± 1.8% |

the estimated confidence intervals for each of the ratios in Table 16-4 compared to those in Table 16-7. The smallest interval in the first set of months is plus or minus 16.6 percent for the small hospital versus plus or minus 3.6 percent for the large. The smallest in the second set is plus or minus 9.3 percent in the small versus plus or minus 1.9 percent in the large. In the third set the best ratio for the small hospital has a confidence range of plus or minus 2.9 percent while the large hospital enjoys a ratio with a range as small as plus or minus 0.7 percent.

The confidence intervals in the two intermediate-sized facilities fall roughly between these two extremes, though the smaller of the two shows slightly greater precision than the larger. Although size is a major determinant of year-to-year variability, it is clearly not the only factor. In general, however, larger facilities can expect earlier precise estimates using this technique than can smaller hospitals.

**Table 16-6** 175-Bed Hospital

| Period | Mean Ratio | Standard Deviation | Estimated Confidence Interval |
|---|---|---|---|
| April | .0812 | .0087 | ± 21.0% |
| May | .0812 | .0039 | ± 9.4% |
| June | .0776 | .0058 | ± 14.7% |
| AM | .1624 | .0117 | ± 14.1% |
| MJ | .1588 | .0097 | ± 12.0% |
| AMJ | .2401 | .0162 | ± 13.2% |
| JJ | .1544 | .0094 | ± 11.9% |
| JJA | .2317 | .0118 | ± 10.0% |
| JJAS | .3121 | .0127 | ± 8.0% |
| MJJ | .2357 | .0103 | ± 8.5% |
| MJJA | .3128 | .0142 | ± 8.8% |
| MJJAS | .3932 | .0180 | ± 9.0% |
| AMJJ | .3170 | .0229 | ± 14.1% |
| AMJJA | .3942 | .0250 | ± 12.4% |
| AMJJAS | .4745 | .0274 | ± 11.3% |
| July | .0769 | .0046 | ± 11.7% |
| JA | .1541 | .0075 | ± 9.5% |
| JAS | .2344 | .0101 | ± 8.4% |
| JASO | .3176 | .0148 | ± 9.1% |
| JASON | .4007 | .0159 | ± 7.8% |
| JASOND | .4815 | .0151 | ± 6.1% |
| JASONDJ | .5733 | .0124 | ± 4.2% |
| JASONDJF | .6585 | .0087 | ± 2.6% |
| JASONDJFM | .7480 | .0098 | ± 2.6% |

## USE OF THE TABLES

There are essentially two ways in which the ratios and standard deviations shown in these tables can be used in decision making. First, early-warning, updated forecasts of the year's utilization can be developed as a basis for considering whether to intervene, given budget estimates and bottom line consequences. Second, the probability of meeting the original utilization forecast can be estimated as a guide to evaluating the risk of not intervening.

To estimate annual utilization for the budget year prior to the year, the April, May, and June ratios would be employed. To obtain the greatest precision, the period with the smallest confidence interval should be selected. In the small hospital (Table 16-4), April by itself offers the most precise estimate (plus or minus 16.6 percent). If April of this year had 700 patient

**Table 16-7** 400-Bed Hospital

| Period | Mean Ratio | Standard Deviation | Estimated Confidence Interval |
|---|---|---|---|
| April | .0870 | .0044 | ± 9.9% |
| May | .0878 | .0027 | ± 6.0% |
| June | .0819 | .0015 | ± 3.6% |
| AM | .1748 | .0065 | ± 7.3% |
| MJ | .1697 | .0032 | ± 5.2% |
| AMJ | .2567 | .0068 | ± 3.7% |
| JJ | .1627 | .0031 | ± 3.7% |
| JJA | .2420 | .0024 | ± 1.9% |
| JJAS | .3211 | .0047 | ± 2.9% |
| MJJ | .2505 | .0052 | ± 4.1% |
| MJJA | .3298 | .0064 | ± 3.8% |
| MJJAS | .4089 | .0065 | ± 3.1% |
| AMJJ | .3375 | .0092 | ± 5.3% |
| AMJJA | .4168 | .0086 | ± 4.0% |
| AMJJAS | .4959 | .0093 | ± 3.7% |
| July | .0808 | .0030 | ± 7.3% |
| JA | .1601 | .0027 | ± 3.3% |
| JAS | .2392 | .0024 | ± 2.0% |
| JASO | .3238 | .0024 | ± 1.5% |
| JASON | .4063 | .0032 | ± 1.5% |
| JASOND | .4852 | .0040 | ± 1.6% |
| JASONDJ | .5740 | .0042 | ± 1.4% |
| JASONDJF | .6543 | .0038 | ± 1.1% |
| JASONDJFM | .7406 | .0027 | ± 0.7% |

days, the early warning forecast for next year would be 700 ÷ .0817 = 8,568 patient days, a projected ADC of 23.5.

For the 105-bed hospital (Table 16-5) the most precise forecast would also be based on April. If it experiences 2,550 patient days during April, it would forecast 2,550 ÷ .0833 = 30,612 patient days, an ADC of 83.9. For the 175-bed facility the month of May offers the best precision. If May had 3,750 patient days, the forecast for the next year would be 3,750 ÷ .0812 = 46,182 patient days, an ADC of 126.5. The large hospital would get roughly the same precision from June alone (plus or minus 3.6 percent) or May and June combined (plus or minus 3.7 percent). If June came in with 10,500 patient days, the forecast would be 10,500 ÷ .0819 = 128,205 patient days, for an ADC of 351.2.

Similar choices would be made as the early months of the budget year pass. Generally, if the confidence interval for the forecast includes the budget utilization level, there could be some confidence that present operations will result in the expected bottom line (assuming revenues and expenditures are also in line). Given the standard deviation of past ratios, the likelihood of annual utilization being at least equal to original estimates, or for that matter not being up to predicted levels, can be calculated based on the normal distribution.

With the 105-bed hospital as an example, if April's utilization is 2,000 patient days and the year's budget is based on 25,500 patient days, the following analysis would be used. With April at 2,000 patient days, the estimate would be 2,000 ÷ .0833 = 24,010 patient days. For the year to be 25,500, April's ratio would have to be 2,000 ÷ 25,500 = .0784. This would be .0833 − .0784 = .0049 below the mean. With a standard deviation of .0041 this would be 1.195 standard deviations below the mean. Based on normal distribution tables, the one-tailed probability of observations 1.195 standard deviations below the mean is .1161. Therefore, the probability of utilization *not* being up to the budget level would be 1.000 − .1161 = .8839, almost 90 percent.

In most cases the exact predicted utilization level need not be achieved in order to realize satisfactory results. In the preceding example as long as annual patient days are at least 25,000 the hospital might be "safe." The probability of achieving at least this minimum utilization would be estimated in similar fashion. With 2,000 patient days in April, annual utilization of 25,000 patient days would mean a ratio of 2,000 ÷ 25,000 = .0800. This would be .0033 below the mean ratio of .0833. With a standard deviation of .0041 this would be .0033 ÷ .0041 = .805 standard deviations below the mean. The chances of such an event would be .2184 according to the normal distribution. Thus the chances are .7816 that annual utilization will be below 25,000 patient days, judging by April's experience.

## DISCUSSION

All these estimates are projections in that they rely on past utilization to forecast utilization. They are also autocorrelations of sorts because they use the relationships between one specific period's utilization and another's to develop the forecast. In any case the technique is naive in not addressing why past ratios have existed or what might cause them to be different in the future. Because the technique is used for immediate-range forecasting, using a naive technique is not the most dangerous choice.

Where there are good reasons to believe that past ratios are not reliable for the present situation, of course, a naive technique should not be relied on. If the hospital or one of its competitors experiences a nurses' strike early in its fiscal year, the ratios for the affected months would probably not be reliable in forecasting the year's utilization unless the strike lasts all year. If specific foreseeable events alter the pattern of utilization experienced early in the year (e.g., arrival of physicians, opening of new services, or closing of a current service), experience would not be a sufficient basis for forecasting.

For example, one of the hospitals used to illustrate this technique experienced significant shifts in local dynamics during the year with significant consequences for annual utilization. The hospital's actual utilization in April, May, and June produced early warning forecasts that the following year's ADC would be right around 136.0, as used in preparing the budget. Some of this utilization, however, represented a one-time surge in use associated with large numbers of layoffs in local industries during the early months of the year. People laid off were taking advantage of the 90-day continuing insurance coverage available to them following loss of employment.

Starting in July, the monthly utilization figures produced new forecasts that consistently hovered around an annual ADC of 124.0, significantly below the 136.0 budget estimate. Effective January 1, a major local insurance group notified physicians that it was experiencing costs well above revenues. If hospital utilization weren't cut back, there wouldn't be enough money available to pay physicians. Beginning in January, local utilization dropped even more dramatically, and early warning estimates began to forecast an annual ADC of 115.0. The year turned out to have an ADC of 115.3.

There was no way that this early warning technique could *anticipate* such developments because it relies on the persistence of past relationships. The hospital had early warning that utilization would probably be well below the budget estimate of a 136.0 ADC, at least. This enabled it to begin cutting expenditures, so that the effect of further declines in utilization over the last six months of the fiscal year would not be as drastic. Familiarity with the local situation and a good understanding of its dynamics should always be preferred to mechanically produced forecasts.

## SUMMARY

Once seasonal variation patterns or cycles are known, they can be used to predict total annual utilization based on early use of specific services. Utilization on Monday may be used to predict what will happen the rest of the week, or utilization on Friday may offer useful insights into what will occur during the following week. All that is necessary is that such fluctuation patterns be consistent in the past for precision and persistent in the future for accuracy.

An example of an actual application of this approach involves the use of monthly inpatient census figures to predict annual inpatient utilization in a group of four hospitals. By accurately measuring the relationships between monthly and annual utilization levels in past years, predictive mean ratios and their standard deviations were identified. These were used individually and in combination to develop early warnings regarding what annual utilization might be in contrast to the expectations used in making budget decisions.

The purpose of these early warnings is to provide the basis for making pro-active management or marketing decisions. The earlier such decisions are made and implemented, the less drastic and more effective they are likely to be. Of course, the earlier the early warning forecasts are made, the less likely they are to be accurate. This produces what is necessarily the classic trade-off problem in forecasting between being sure of the forecast and being early enough with a decision to optimize its effect.

**Part VI**

# Forecasting Applications

The chapters in this final part of the book are designed to illustrate how forecasting thoughts and techniques can be used in specific decision contexts. If any point worth making is worth belaboring, then this part reaffirms the author's contention that forecasts are only as good as the decisions that they guide and facilitate. For all but hobby forecasters who are not involved with making any decisions, these chapters should provide insights into what to do with forecasts and how to develop them in the most useful manner.

Chapter 17 addresses the use of utilization forecasts in making decisions in general. It discusses in some detail one of the most useful adjuncts to forecasting: sensitivity analysis and the five forms of this analytical tool that are useful in using forecasts to make decisions. A model identifying the interaction of forecasts and decisions in the success of a decision is presented. Specific consequences of decisions are discussed as the basis for making the best decision in light of forecast use of health services.

Chapter 18 discusses one of the most difficult challenges to forecasting: estimating the use of a proposed service or program. Both use of a new service in general and use of a specific provider are discussed together with specific forecasting techniques appropriate for each. Three illustrations of this challenge are given: forecasting use of a new kidney dialysis program, inpatient utilization for a new hospital, and visits to a new primary care center. The basic guidelines and techniques appropriate to these three examples cover essentially all the new service utilization situations likely to arise.

# Chapter 17

# Forecasting and Decision Making

The focus of all previous chapters has been on forecasting use of health services. Decisions should be made not on the basis of future utilization, however, but on the *effects* of such utilization. While utilization has been the effect, and forecasting has focused on what causes it to change in previous discussions, decision making must concern itself with what effects different levels of utilization cause.

Fortunately the techniques described for forecasting utilization, with the exception of projections, can be used to forecast the impact of utilization on whatever values are held to be important in making a decision. Any of the prediction techniques can be used to forecast effects, with utilization as the predictive factor. There should be, in most cases, well-known, quantitative relationships between utilization and efficiency, revenues, expenses, staffing requirements, for example.

Where clear quantitative relationships are not known, a Delphi or judgment process can be used to estimate effects of utilization. Impacts on the health of the community, for example, probably can only be estimated in this fashion, though analogs from previous experience may also serve. Whatever values are pertinent to the decision should be amenable to forecasting as consequences of whatever utilization levels are forecast.

If the *type* of utilization has significant impact on values pertinent to the decision, then utilization by type would have to be forecast. Patient mix for utilization would arise from utilization forecasts by service population or market segment. The consequences of utilization by patient type may be forecast as revenues if patient mix is in terms of payment source; as staffing needs if by acuity level or diagnosis; and as accommodation requirements if by inpatient service, for example. Whatever consequences are to be used in making a decision should be predictable based on the utilization forecasts.

## SENSITIVITY ANALYSIS

In using a forecast for making a decision, there should be some level or range of utilization at which a decision would change. This applies to all discrete decisions, i.e., where the action to be taken is whether or not to do something. Where the decision is of a continuous nature, involving how much or how many, the decision would presumably alter for each utilization forecast shift.

Forecast sensitivity analysis begins by substituting two or more levels of utilization within the range of forecast possibilities to see if different decisions would result. Typically the low, high, and midpoint of the range of utilization likely for the future would be used. If the decision makers conclude that the same decision would be made for each of these different utilization levels, then that decision is *insensitive* to the uncertainty associated with the forecast, and things are simple.

In many cases, however, the decision would differ for different utilization forecasts, either from a yes to a no discrete decision or from some level to another in a semidiscrete decision such as building a hospital with one, two, or three nursing units or an office building with one, two, or three stories. Where substantially different decisions would be made depending on which level in the range of forecast utilization were relied on, then the decision is sensitive to the uncertainty of the forecast, and more work is needed.

Most likely the determination of what decision makes sense relative to different levels of utilization is based on the anticipated (i.e., forecast) impact of utilization on the organization's success. Different levels of utilization mean different revenue, expense, perhaps even quality, and certainly different impact on health. There is likely to be some minimum amount of utilization necessary to justify whatever investment of time, effort, and resources would attend the decision.

Where there is a clear sensitivity point or range where a decision would change and where forecast utilization levels straddle the sensitive area, then the forecast is insufficiently precise. At this point there are two possible responses. The decision makers may choose to gamble based on estimated probabilities of utilization being equal to or below the sensitivity level. If uncomfortable about the gamble, they may seek to refine the forecast so as to improve its precision. This does not remove the risk, of course, because all forecasts of utilization are uncertain, but it may build greater confidence in the decision.

In addition to forecasting sensitivity, there are a number of other areas in which sensitivity analysis applies in decision making. The essence of sensitivity is the substitution of reasonably likely alternative values. If this substitution occurs in the utilization forecast, it applies as described previously, as a *forecast sensitivity analysis*. If substitution occurs in the factors used to develop the forecast in the first place, it is *causal sensitivity analysis*. When it is applied to the outcomes or consequences of the forecast, it is *outcome sensitivity analysis*. When it is used relative to decision criteria, it is *criteria sensitivity analysis*. When it is applied to the decision itself, it is *decision sensitivity analysis*.

**Causal Sensitivity**

Sensitivity analysis applied to causal or predictive factors used in developing a forecast of utilization has two uses. First, it can be used to reexamine a forecast of utilization in terms of whether forecasts of what is happening to or measurements of the status of causal factors are acceptable. Second, it can be used to select specific factors for attention in order to employ marketing strategies to ensure a forecast utilization level.

Reexamination of a utilization forecast based on estimates of the present or future status of causal factors first identifies which factors have the greatest impact on the forecast. In forecasting hospital utilization, for example, the size of the population or its age mix might be the most important factors. These would be identified through examination of standardized beta values and comparison of the mathematical contribution of individual independent variables if a multiple linear regression had been used to develop the forecast. If a prospection technique such as change factor forecasting were employed, the percentage change contribution made by each factor would be used to select the highest impacts.

Once the most critical factors are identified, i.e., those to which the forecast of utilization was most sensitive, forecasters reexamine each factor. The first question asked is whether there is any doubt about the present status of the factor if a time-lagged forecast is used or about its estimated future status where time lagging is not involved. Recognizing the importance of a population forecast, for example, is the forecast used the best one available? If it were supplied by an outside agency, what is the track record of that agency? If its 1975 estimate of the 1980 population were off 10 percent, can forecasters of utilization rely on its 1985 forecast of 1990 population?

The method used to develop estimates of the present or future status of a significant factor should be examined more carefully when it is discovered that the utilization forecast is particularly sensitive to it. Would different assumptions have led to significantly different estimates? Is there more uncertainty in the estimate than reflected in the way the utilization forecast was developed? Are other estimates more likely?

By substituting alternative values for critical predictive factors, forecasters can mathematically determine how dependent their utilization forecast is on the estimated status of each factor. If the population were 10,000 more or less than the specific estimate used, what difference would it make to the utilization forecast? If the proportion of aged were one percent more or less than the estimate used, what difference would that make?

In addition to postulating alternative estimates for causal factors, forecasters should reexamine the relationship between the predictive or independent variables and utilization, the dependent variable. What would happen to the utilization forecast if the mathematical relationship between population and utilization, i.e., the use rate, varied plus or minus 1 or 2 percent from the value used in prediction? How likely is some shift in this relationship?

Asking these sensitivity questions is simply a form of second-guessing ourselves relative to forecasting. If we answer the questions with renewed confidence in original estimates, then we gain greater confidence in the forecast. If we recognize uncertainty that somehow was overlooked in the original forecast, we may take greater care to improve that forecast or be more flexible in our decision, with good preparation for contingencies. In either case we should feel better about the decision.

Potentially more useful in causal sensitivity analysis are cases where the critical causal factors are subject to direct manipulation or influence by forecasters. Population and age mix would be strictly passive factors in most cases. By contrast the number of physicians in the community, the prices for specific services, even people's attitudes toward a given service or provider can certainly be influenced. If one of these or similarly influenceable variables turn out to be critical in forecasting utilization— and if a decision is sensitive to a specific level of utilization—causal sensitivity analysis can be used to select the factors to be employed in deliberate marketing efforts.

The technique is the same for influenceable as well as passive predictive factors. Alternative values of critical factors are selected to test how sensitive the utilization forecast is to reasonably achievable states of each. If adding one physician would shift the utilization forecast upward or downward significantly, recruitment of such a physician might be considered. The *value* of such an increase in utilization, given the decision, can be used to determine how much could reasonably be spent in a recruitment effort. If such a recruitment appears unlikely to succeed or would involve more expense than its value to the organization, the decision might be altered accordingly.

**Outcome Sensitivity**

Outcome sensitivity treats the utilization forecast as the causal or predictive factor, and one or more specific success criteria as consequences thereof. The purpose of this analysis is first to determine the difference in performance outcomes or program success if utilization were slightly more or less than forecast. How much would a 1 or 2 percent variation in utilization affect revenues, expenses, and profit, for example? Could utilization quite reasonably be 1 or 2 percent more or less than originally forecast?

The technique for outcome sensitivity analysis is the same as for all forms of this analysis. Substitute values for utilization levels are used to generate hypothetical outcome or performance levels. If changes in utilization tend to have significant impact on performance, enough to make a difference in the decision to be made, then a reexamination of the utilization forecast is called for. If by chance a reasonable shift from the original utilization forecast has no significant effect on performance, this would reinforce the decision based on the original forecast.

If the decision is sensitive to the range of outcomes resulting from slightly different levels of utilization, two steps are called for. First is reexamination of the utilization forecast. Are slightly different levels of utilization likely? Can we do anything to increase the likelihood of utilization being at the "right" level in terms of the decision? By knowing the value of increasing utilization in terms of performance outcomes, we can determine how much it's worth to do so. Second, we should reexamine the relationship between utilization and performance. Would slightly different utilization levels really alter performance outcomes as originally predicted? Given fixed and variable costs, would financial outcomes really be as good or bad as first thought?

**Criteria Sensitivity**

Criteria sensitivity analysis substitutes alternative success criteria or outcomes relative to a given utilization forecast and decision to see if they make any difference. If different performance outcomes were considered, or given different weights, would a different conclusion be reached? If financial return were downgraded in importance, for example, would the decision change for a given utilization forecast? If consideration of the needs of the community for service or the costs to them of seeking care elsewhere were added to decision criteria, would that alter the decision?

By reexamining the impact specific criteria have on a decision, given the level of utilization forecast, decision makers can test their own sensitivity to those criteria. If a financial criterion makes the difference between a yes or no decision, does the organization truly wish to rely completely on financial considerations? Are financial consequences so highly valued by the organization, such a dominant motivation, that they should dictate the decision? Conversely, if financial considerations were raised slightly in importance, would the decision shift from yes to no? If so, can the organization afford to absorb poor financial consequences in light of whatever other criteria justified a yes decision?

**Decision Sensitivity**

The final form of sensitivity analysis postulates alternative *decisions* to see if outcomes would be different for a given utilization forecast. If additional treatment rooms were designed into a clinic, could utilization volumes be handled with lower staff costs, hence produce more favorable financial outcomes? If the clinic operated more days each week or more hours per day, could utilization volumes be accommodated with less space and equipment costs? Even though this might add to personnel costs, might this alter the performance enough to suggest that the decision should be changed?

In general, the way to make any decision is to forecast the consequences of alternative decisions in terms of performance outcomes or success criteria for the organization. Decision sensitivity analysis calls on decision makers to use their imaginations in postulating reasonable alternative decisions to be considered. By examining consequences of a large number in light of the forecast of utilization arrived at, the "best" decision should be found, rather than merely a satisfactory one.

**Combined Sensitivity Analysis**

With computer capacity it is relatively simple to combine all forms of sensitivity analysis for a given decision. Programs can be written to substitute hypothetical but reasonable alternatives for all the values used in making a decision:

- predictive factors used to forecast utilization
- utilization levels
- performance outcomes
- success criteria
- decisions

Ideally such analysis finds relatively low sensitivity:

- Utilization forecasts do not change much in response to small variations in predictive factors.
- Performance outcomes do not change much in response to small variations in utilization or alternative decisions.
- Decisions would not differ much in response to slight changes in utilization, performance impacts, or success criteria.

If hypothetical manipulations of the factors in making the ultimate decision do not produce significant differences, great confidence can be placed in the decision. Where significant sensitivity to changes in predictive factors, utilization levels, performance outcomes, success criteria, or decisions is noted, decision makers have two basic choices. More careful consideration can be given to the values for each of these components in the decision process in order to yield a higher level of confidence in one versus another decision. If there is not time for more analysis or it produces no result, ultimately a gamble must be taken and a decision made in spite of significant uncertainty. In any forecasting situation, uncertainty is unavoidable; there is always a matter of the degree of risk rather than its elimination.

- Causal sensitivity analysis substitutes hypothetical values for predictive factors to see what differences result in utilization forecasts.
- Forecast sensitivity analysis substitutes hypothetical values for utilization levels to see what differences result in outcomes.
- Outcome sensitivity analysis substitutes hypothetical values for outcomes to see what differences result in final decision.
- Criteria sensitivity analysis substitutes different sets of outcomes or gives them different weights to see what differences result in final decision.
- Decision sensitivity analysis substitutes different decisions to see if different performance outcomes result.

As the model in Figure 17-1 indicates, the dynamics of the "rational" decision process are predicated on a number of forecasts. Given what we expect of developments in causal or predictive factors, what utilization do we expect? Given utilization and any given decision or given a decision and any given utilization, what performance do we expect? Given performance, what shall our final decision be? Sensitivity analysis forms examine how differences in one or more of the components of these dynamics might

**Figure 17-1** Model of Sensitivity Analysis

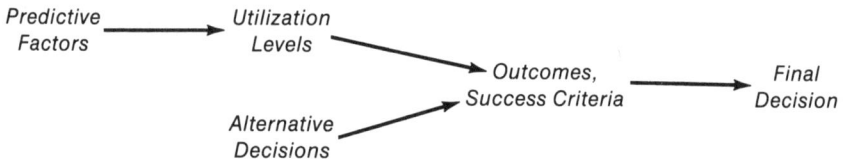

Predictive ──────────▶ Utilization
Factors                 Levels ──────────▶ Outcomes, ──────────▶ Final
                                            Success Criteria        Decision
                        Alternative ──────▶
                        Decisions

lead to a different decision. The forecasting of developments and consequences is only as good as the decision that is made and its effect on the organization.

## SUCCESS CRITERIA CONSEQUENCES

In order to employ utilization forecasts to make the best decisions, it is first necessary to have in mind the kinds of success criteria or performance outcomes that will be affected by utilization. Such criteria or important outcomes are likely to be idiosyncratic to each health care organization. However, it is still possible to list and discuss the kinds of criteria that might apply, to differing extents and with differing importance, to organizations making decisions based on utilization forecasts.

### Financial Consequences

The most obvious outcome area is financial. Utilization levels have specific and predictable consequences on revenues and expenditures, hence on profit and organizational viability. Given fixed versus variable costs, the consequences of utilization relative to expenses require special care in forecasting. For many services this is equally true for income because different *types* of patients pay widely different amounts based on their insurance coverage, eligibility for government reimbursement, deductible and copayment requirements, eligibility for charitable care, and ability and willingness to make payment.

Forecasting utilization of services by a population is only the first step in predicting financial consequences. Models of expenditure links to utilization and different design features of a program are needed to estimate expenditure consequences. Forecasts of the specific mix of patients by diagnosis and acuity level may be needed to predict total expenditures. The mix of patients by payment source and subsequently by diagnosis and acuity level may be needed to predict the income consequences of utilization. Both expenditure and income forecasts are obviously needed to estimate profitability of specific operations and reach specific design or basic program decisions.

## Quality Consequences

Unless the organization is in business entirely to make profits and is insensitive to other performance outcomes, criteria such as the quality consequences of utilization are likely to be important. It has been shown in numerous studies that for high-technology, sophisticated services, quality tends to increase with utilization volumes. It takes a certain amount of practice for individual providers and teams to acquire and maintain high-skill levels. This translates into differences in expected complications, mortality, malpractice suits, and other real, quantifiable, and significant quality measures.

By the same token there are bound to be utilization volumes, relative to capacity, that are too high to maintain optimum quality. Utilization that overcrowds physical space or overtaxes personnel is obviously likely to affect quality adversely. Whether the effects of too high utilization levels will show up in mortality or complications is not so clear as when utilization levels are too low. Nevertheless specific, real, and quantifiable effects in terms of patient transfers in hospitals, readmission rates resulting from too early discharge, and others should certainly be expected and watched for.

## Efficiency Consequences

Any organization delivering health care can only be as efficient as its utilization permits. Once space is developed, equipment purchased, personnel hired, and materials bought, the capacity of the organization to provide care is given. How efficiently that capacity is used is then a function of how many people use how many services. Thus efficiency is not merely a measure of management performance; it is certainly a reflection of marketing performance as well.

Management enters into efficiency whenever it can make alternative decisions relative to capacity. Unfortunately such decisions often must be made well in advance (lead time) and have lasting, almost permanent consequences (duration) as discussed in Chapter 2. Once made, some correction and adjustments may be possible. For the most part, however, efficiency is affected more by marketing success than management manipulations.

## Convenience

Utilization levels relative to capacity have a lot to do with the ability of the organization to offer convenience of service to its markets. Volumes of patient demand on a physician's office, clinic, ambulatory care program, hospital, or long-term care facility affect whether patients can be cared for immediately or must wait and how long. In turn the convenience offered by a given provider can determine whether people are treated in a timely fashion (quality) and how they feel about service (satisfaction). The satisfaction levels can then influence utilization by patients, their families, and acquaintances.

A complex interaction exists between convenience and utilization. It amounts to what is termed *negative feedback loop* in systems dynamics (Chapter 8). A new program can offer excellent convenience, immediate appointments, and little or no waiting time. As it becomes more successful, however, and utilization increases, the ability to offer such convenience naturally diminishes. With decreasing convenience, satisfaction tends to decline, and utilization decreases. With lower utilization, convenience should increase again, with higher satisfaction and growing utilization until the cycle repeats.

Because the capacity of a program, measured in terms of space, equipment, and personnel, is adjustable only in substantial and infrequent increments, it is difficult to offer constant convenience. This problem tends to be worse the smaller the program is. As medical care providers and programs move into more sparsely populated areas, this reality greatly affects the competitive success of specific programs. Substantial fluctuations in utilization levels from year to year should be expected and managed as a natural phenomenon in programs serving smaller populations.

## Contribution

For any health care program motivated by the desire to make a significant contribution to the health of its community, utilization is the major determinant of how great a contribution it can make. This is true in two separate but related ways. First, the volume of utilization reflects the sheer numbers of people reached by the organization, hence the numbers to which it can make a contribution. Second, whether people use the organization's service as often and consistently as they should determines the extent of that contribution.

Because these performance outcomes or success criteria may conflict with each other, utilization forecasts may lead to appropriately different decisions by different organizations. In some cases the contribution made by a given level of utilization justifies offering a program even though financial consequences are below par. Quality considerations may suggest refraining from offering a service even though expected utilization volumes may be financially promising.

Even with a given decision, specific management responses to utilization can have conflicting performance consequences. Capacity decisions designed to maximize efficiency and minimize expenditures can significantly reduce convenience and vice versa. Efforts to enhance quality, given utilization levels, may add to expenditures and reduce efficiency.

Utilization given any decision, or any decision given utilization, produces specific performance consequences. In making any decision based on utilization forecasts, the expected performance consequences on whatever success criteria the organization values should be considered. Many of the forecasting techniques described in this book are potential choices for predicting. Essentially any technique that employs a predictive relationship, whether through mathematical analysis or informed judgment, is an option. The considerations appropriate for determining which is preferred in forecasting utilization, i.e., consistency and expected persistence of relationships, are equally appropriate for deciding how to forecast its consequences. A decision will turn out well when and because both the forecast utilization and its consequences turn out as expected or close enough.

## SUMMARY

The purpose for developing forecasts of utilization is to make good decisions; it is the decision that determines how good the forecast is. In turn, what determines the effectiveness of the decision is what impact it has on the organization, given the utilization. In examining alternative decisions, utilization and those decisions are independent, predictive variables, and their joint consequences are the dependent or outcome variables in a forecasting process. Thus, any of the causally oriented prediction and prospection techniques discussed as tools for forecasting utilization can be used to forecast consequences of decisions.

In considering alternative decisions in light of utilization expectations, it is useful to examine the extent to which a final decision might be altered if one or more of the estimated or forecast realities used to reach that decision were different. The technique of sensitivity analysis is used to carry out such an examination.

Five types of sensitivity analysis are useful in decision making: (1) forecast, (2) causal, (3) outcome, (4) criteria, and (5) decision sensitivity analysis. Each substitutes hypothetical but reasonably likely alternatives for the values used in reaching the original decision. If such substitutions fail to dislodge the original decision as clearly preferred, then that decision is insensitive to such alternatives, and decision makers can feel great confidence in the appropriateness of that decision. If the decision would be substantially different, even opposite the original, if something were slightly different, then the decision is sensitive to the difference.

If sensitivity is established to one or more of the five inputs to the decision process, decision makers should reexamine the original inputs to determine whether they should reconsider the decision. In some cases reexamination clearly either confirms or changes the original input. If so, this should be reflected through reaffirming or changing the final decision. If further consideration still leaves doubt, however, then the decision makers must take whatever gamble they feel is most appropriate. When dealing with the future, gambling should be accepted as a natural necessity.

**Annotated Bibliography**

Aderholdt, J. "A Valuable Key to Financial Feasibility Studies for Hospitals." *Hospital Financial Management* 34, no. 9 (September 1981):52.

Clark, B., and Lamont, G. "Accurate Census Forecasting Leads to Cost Containment." *Hospitals,* June 1, 1976, p. 43.
Describes use of daily census forecasts over a one-year period to achieve optimum occupancy of staffed beds, optimum personnel expenditures, fewer admission cancellations, accurate revenue projections, and efficient cleaning and renovation schedules.

Cleverly, W. "Profitability Analysis in the Hospital Industry." *Health Services Research* 13, no. 1 (Spring 1978):16.
Discusses how utilization levels in the future affect the profitability of specific hospital decisions, hence dictate which decisions are reasonable.

Donlon, V. "Statistical Methods to Forecast Volume of Services for the Revenue Budget." *Hospital Financial Management* 34, no. 3 (March 1983):83.
Discusses the use of forecasts in making decisions regarding hospital charges.

Fetter, R., and Thompson, J. "A Planning Model for the Delivery of Health Services." Chap. 13 in *Health Care Delivery Planning,* edited by A. Reisman and M. Kiley. New York; Gordon Breach, 1973, p. 302.
Describes ways of predicting consumption of specific resources as a function of health services use.

Gardner, E., and McLaughlin, C. "Forecasting: A Cost Control Tool for Health Care Managers." *Health Care Management Review* 5, no. 3 (Summer 1980):31.
Describes how to employ forecasts of utilization to plan and control hospital expenditures.

Long, H. "Valuation as a Criterion in Not-for-Profit Decision Making." *Health Care Management Review* 1, no. 3 (Summer 1976).
Discusses ways to estimate the value impact of specific alternative decisions.

**Warner, M., et al.** ''A Strategic Planning Model for Multihospital Systems.'' *Inquiry* 18, no. 3 (Fall 1981):214.
   Describes a model used to predict financial performance of hospitals based on diagnostic-specific utilization forecasts.

# Chapter 18

# Forecasting Use of New Services

A frequent challenge with health services is the forecasting of utilization for a new service. Forecasts may first be needed to enable the organization to decide whether to offer such a program and to design specific capacity and features of the program if it is to be offered. Even after satisfying itself, if the decision is to go ahead, the organization may have to develop additional forecasts for financial feasibility studies or regulatory approval. Pro forma financial statements are generated on the basis of utilization levels. The "need" for a given program is evaluated at least partly on the basis of expected utilization.

In forecasting use of a new service, two separate forecasts are needed. First, the forecast of the *total market* for a given service must be developed. The total market represents all the people who might reasonably use the service and all the use that they might reasonably make of that service, assuming that it were available. Second is the *market share* of any given provider competitive to any and all other providers. The combination of the total market times a provider's share is the utilization that any specific provider may enjoy.

## TOTAL MARKET

The total amount of utilization available for a given provider to share is a function of two separate components. First is the utilization that results from the natural service population in a given area. Depending on the specific service, the natural service population may be people living within a few miles, in a city or county, throughout a major metropolitan area, or in a vast region extending even beyond state boundaries.

The natural service area for a given service is partly a function of the psychographics of the physician and patient population, partly a function of the access afforded by providers, and partly a function of the number and location of other providers. In turn, access and competition are significantly affected by the potential market, the costs, and income potential of the service. There is absolutely no simple formula or technique for identifying the natural service area for a given service, nor is it possible to define such an area permanently in practice. Informed judgment and an awareness of the possibility of change are required.

Psychographics affect service areas in that the distance and difficulty of obtaining a specific service affect whether physicians refer patients or patients seek the service in the first place. Depending on the *necessity* of the service as perceived by physician, patient, and family compared to the travel cost, price, difficulty plus any negative consequences of traveling to the nearest appropriate source, a given person may or may not be in the market. As the numbers of providers increase, the *total* market for utilization of a given service also tends to increase, though the natural service area for a specific provider is likely to diminish, to say nothing of its market share.

The choice of a natural service area is primarily one of practical logic, because it determines the sort of analysis and consideration that follows. Once the natural market is identified and its potential utilization determined, the task is to determine how much of that natural market is retained by providers serving the market. The second task is to estimate the number of people who will use services offered by these providers even though those people live outside the natural market. This inflow normally represents a small but significant portion of the total local market in which a given provider might share.

The combination of retention and inflow adds up to the total local market. If there is only one provider in that market, the forecast of its utilization is simply this sum. If there is more than one provider in the area, a further forecast must be made of the share to be enjoyed by each. The size of the natural market should be determined so that it represents the vast majority of the potential market, 80 percent to 95 percent of the total in most cases. Inflow is forecast using a lower level of analysis and less information, so should not represent too large a proportion of the total.

From a practical perspective the natural service area should be defined in such a way as to facilitate obtaining useful data. If utilization forecasts are to be based primarily on psychographic information such as perceived health status or interest, the service area may be defined in terms of zip codes or telephone prefixes, depending on whether telephone interviews or mailed questionnaires are to be used in gathering data. If demographic data are needed, units available for such data, i.e., census tracts, cities, counties, states, and regions, make sense. If physicians are the primary market, either their office locations or homes may make up the basic service area.

## NEED

The total local market size is first a function of the need for a given service. If a new program is intended to serve all those suffering from a specific condition, then epidemiological data regarding the incidence and prevalence of the condition should be sought. Local health departments, disease registries, and medical groups are the logical sources of such information. Associations that raise money for research and treatment of specific diseases may also have data but usually not firsthand. Physicians and other professionals treating the disease and organizations of people suffering from the disease and their families may also be sources of data.

Need does not represent the full size of the market, however. All people who might benefit from a given service because of having a specific disease or condition represent the total need for a service. Not all such people recognize their status, however, and some may perceive themselves in need when they are not. For any service based on diagnosing disease or condition, demand for diagnosis includes some portion of all people truly having that disease or condition plus some number of people erroneously believing themselves to have it.

Diagnosis demand therefore is some percentage of need plus a number without need. This is mathematically equivalent to retention and inflow. In other words, if total "need," i.e., people having a specific need or condition, is 10,000 people, 80 percent might recognize their status and seek care. This amounts to 8,000 people. In addition, depending on how well known symptoms are, how concerned people are about them, and how much faith they have in medical care, there may be other thousands of people seeking care. In the case of a cardiac care unit, for example, large numbers of people present themselves or are brought to emergency rooms with symptoms of possible heart attack and are diagnosed for something entirely different. This additional demand might be anywhere from a small number to a number greater than the appropriate demand.

This "rule-out" demand that needs merely to be diagnosed and eliminated from subsequent treatment demand should be forecast separately from "true" demand. It is always possible to calculate it as a proportion of true demand or of total demand, but this is not a valid method to forecast it. The factors affecting spurious demand are simply not the same as those affecting true demand, so they should not be forecast as having a constant relationship. Efforts are often appropriate either to increase false demand in order to reach more people who really do suffer a given disease or condition or to decrease it in order to eliminate wasteful use of services.

The total service population times the proportion likely to use care represents the total local market for a given service. If the service is brand-new and never before available, demand may be forecast entirely on the basis of estimated need, adjusted for nonresponse by those in need and overresponse by those not in need. If the service substitutes for a previous method of diagnosis or treatment, total demand may be forecast on the basis of use of the existing service. If the new service is significantly superior, it may well draw away virtually all preexisting demand. Additional demand might arise due to superiority if it reflects the new service being safer, more effective, or less expensive.

Some combination of objective analysis and subjective judgment is appropriate for forecasting demand for a new service. Available data regarding the number of people potentially benefiting from the service are a good start. Data on people currently using a service for which the new one would substitute are another. Analogs from other areas where the new service has been introduced represent another source of input. Epidemiological estimates of disease incidence and prevalence constitute yet another source. All such sources may usefully be examined.

What must be kept in mind, however, is that demand for health services is a human behavior. It reflects how potential patients, their families, and physicians react to situations. Perceiving the benefit of a new service may come easily and sweep the local service area in a matter of days or weeks, or it may take years. Spurious demand may be small or large and might be appropriately discouraged or encouraged, depending on the situation.

Forecasting initial response to a new service by a given service population should be based on asking and answering a series of questions:

- What numbers or proportions of the total population would potentially benefit from the service? (Examine data on incidence and prevalence of condition.)

- What numbers or proportions of those potentially benefiting will recognize their situation and seek diagnosis? (Consider how clear symptoms are, how serious people perceive the condition to be, how much faith they have in the efficacy of available treatment.)

- What numbers or proportions of the *total population* will mistakenly perceive themselves as in need and seek care? (Same considerations as in question 2.)

- If demand for treatment is to be forecast, what numbers or proportions of question 2 will be referred for or given treatment? (Consider geographic, cost, and psychological barriers to care.)
- For each person referred for treatment, how many treatments will each receive per year? (Consider recommended number adjusted for missed appointments, lack of compliance, etc.)

Delphi approaches may prove useful in addition to examination of data in answering each of these five questions. In general, the newer, more distinctly different the service from what has been available, the more judgment is required. Where a service replaces something, total demand may be forecast on the basis of recorded existing behavior, but judgment is still needed to forecast the extent and timing of switching from old to new.

## KIDNEY DIALYSIS FORECAST

To illustrate, consider the problem of forecasting demand for a proposed new kidney dialysis program in a community where none had been available. The potential service population for such a program would logically be all those people living closer in travel time and distance to the new program than to other existing programs. The area circumscribed by lines of equal distance between the new program and the nearest alternative should outline the service area. People living within that area are the natural service population. Because of the frequency of dialysis, people tend to use the nearest source, so inflow should be low and retention high.

The starting point in forecasting use of a new kidney dialysis program is identifying the number of people receiving dialysis in the service area. All future utilization begins from this number, based on additions to and subtractions from the number being served. If, at the beginning of a given year, 36 people are receiving dialysis, of whom 20 are treated in a center and 16 at home, this is the numerical starting point. Because there is an expected mortality among such patients, this must be applied to determine the number expected to be receiving dialysis at the end of the year. For illustration, let us use a mortality rate of 10 percent. Of the 20 center patients, 2 would be expected to die during the year and 18 survive. (Because of the small numbers involved, actual deaths may be something other than 2 but would be unpredictable as to whether more or less.)

During the year new cases will arise. If the service population is 200,000 and the incidence rate 60 per million, there would be $200,000 \times .00006 = 12$ new cases expected during the year. If 20% of these have transplants, of which half fail, then .5 × .20 = 10% will not be dialysis clients, i.e., 10% of 12 = 1.2 expected, leaving 10.8 for dialysis. If 40% of the dialysis patients are treated at home, then only 60% of 10.8 = 6.48 would be new center dialysis patients. With a mortality rate of 10%, some of these new patients will not survive the year. Because new cases arise randomly throughout the year, each is at risk of mortality for an expected average of only six months. Thus the expected mortality for new cases would be only 5%. With 95% surviving, there should be .95 × 6.48 = 6.16 new cases by the end of the year. Adding these new cases to the 18 surviving old cases would mean a total of 24.16 at the end of the reference year.

To obtain a forecast of total utilization of dialysis during the year, two figures must be developed. First is the average caseload during the year, and second is the average number of dialysis treatments per case per year. The average caseload is simply the midpoint between the beginning caseload and the year-end figure because new cases and deaths are presumed to occur randomly throughout the year. With 20 center dialysis patients at the beginning of the year and 24.16 at the end, the average caseload would be (20 + 24.16) ÷ 2 = 22.08.

To determine average treatments per patient, the standard case pattern should be applied. If the typical patient receives three dialysis treatments per week, this amounts to 3 × 52 = 156 per year. With an average caseload of 22.08 there would be 22.08 × 156 = 3,444 treatments at the center per year.

To forecast utilization during the next year, a new starting figure of 24.16 would be used. Of these, 10 percent would be expected to be lost, leaving .90 × 24.16 = 21.74. If next year's population is expected to be 205,000, new cases should be 205,000 × .00006 = 12.3. If 10 percent are removed from dialysis due to successful transplants, .90 × 12.3 = 11.07 would remain. If 40 percent of these are treated at home, then .60 × 11.07 = 6.64 would be added to the center caseload. Because only 95 percent would survive the year, this would add .95 × 6.64 = 6.31 to actual cases.

Adding the surviving old cases of 21.74 to the expected surviving new cases of 6.31 would yield a year-end caseload of 21.74 + 6.31 = 28.05. The average caseload for the year would be (24.16 + 28.05) ÷ 2 = 26.1. The annual number of treatments should be 26.1 × 156 = 4,072.

This technique for forecasting utilization applies to existing centers as well as new ones. It also applies to use of any service that fits the incidence and prevalence pattern of end-stage renal disease. Use of cancer treatment, hypertension care, diabetes, or any chronic condition whose incidence rate, initial prevalence, and mortality are known can be predicted in this way. Kidney dialysis is a complex example because of the different forms of treatment available (transplant versus dialysis, home versus center) but is a simpler example because

- almost all patients needing care get it;
- few patients not needing care seek it; and
- market share among competing providers is rarely a problem; choice is dominated by distance when care is sought 156 times per year.

This technique can also be used to forecast utilization of services offered by an HMO. The prevalence figure is the number of enrollees at the beginning of the year. Incidence represents new enrollment. Mortality equals disenrollment either by choice at annual openings (applies to old enrollees only) or due to changing employment (applies to both old and new). Once the incidence, prevalence, and mortality figures are determined, the average caseload for the year can be forecast. This times average utilization per member per year becomes the forecast for the year's total utilization.

Special adjustments might have to be made for unique patterns of use that apply to the first year of enrollment. Such patterns should be adjusted for the expectation that the average new enrollee spends only half the year in the program. The rest of the pattern should be carried over into the subsequent year. If new enrollees are expected to differ in terms of risk, age, etc., from the average, further adjustments might be necessary.

## INPATIENT UTILIZATION FORECAST

Forecasting the use of a specific hospital, whether a year in advance or more, involves anticipating reasonable values for a number of mathematical factors:

- the number of people in its natural service area
- their use of inpatient care
- their likelihood of receiving care with the service area (retention)
- their preference for the specific hospital (market share)
- the numbers of people coming to the hospital from outside the area (inflow)

**Service Population**

The service area population changes modestly from year to year in most cases but may change significantly over a multi-year period. Forecasts of this population may be derived from state government; local city, county, or councils of government; chambers of commerce; utility companies, universities; or any number of sources. The methods and assumptions used by these sources, together with their past track records, should provide some basis for deciding which forecasts are likely to be more reliable. If all seem equally likely, an average of all might be used, but rarely are all equally likely.

The size and age mix of the service population should be forecast in order to provide the basis for anticipating its use of inpatient care. Fine breakdowns of age cohorts are probably not needed for 1- or 2-year forecasts but would be useful for 5, 10, or more years ahead. Changes in age mix should be anticipated because of their significant impact on use rates. The size of the population is always the most significant determinant of utilization.

**Use Rates**

Aside from age mix a host of other factors may influence use rates. Even in the short run a decline in the economy such as in 1980–1983 can significantly depress use rates due to lack of insurance coverage and reluctance to have elective procedures done. Shifts in technology can greatly influence use of specific types of care but rarely have major impact on overall utilization.

In general it is better to predict use of inpatient care by major service categories rather than overall. Factors that determine use of medical, surgical, obstetric, and psychiatric care tend to differ from each other. Pediatric utilization is largely a function of the size of the younger population, especially the 0 to 1 age cohort, which is in turn a function of obstetric utilization. In addition to offering generally superior forecasts of total utilization, using service-specific use rates also leads to better estimates of market share and inflow because these are also susceptible to service-specific change factors.

Use rates should also be broken down into admissions and length of stay because factors affecting these two components are substantially different. By disaggregating use rates into five services and two components, the forecasting challenge requires 10 individual forecasts. Although this complicates the task, it improves both the accuracy and usefulness of the results.

Forecasting surgical utilization, for example, might take into account hospital-sponsored efforts to increase preadmission testing that would reduce length of stay or ambulatory surgery that would reduce admissions. New technology might be expected to simplify some surgeries (e.g., ultrasound disintegration of kidney stones) and reduce length of stay accordingly. Other new procedures might be foreseen to enable surgical intervention where it was not possible before (e.g., coronary bypass), producing a number of new admissions. Conversely new drugs might replace surgery, shifting admissions from surgical to medical in a number of cases.

## Retention

The probability that residents of a defined service area will seek and receive hospital care within that area varies widely with circumstances. For suburban areas with a few local hospitals offering modest programs, close to a major metropolitan medical complex, retention may be less than 50 percent in many cases. As suburban hospitals grow and add specialized services, this retention tends to increase and can easily reach 60 to 75 percent. In intermediate cities, far from major urban centers but with most basic specialties available, retention in the range of 75 to 90 percent is not unreasonable. In isolated rural areas, with only primary level services available and within reasonable distance of referral centers, 50 to 65 percent may be typical.

There is absolutely no *rule,* however, regarding what retention should be or will be in any particular case. Retention can be increased by any individual hospital simply by expanding capacity and adding services. Often retention is enhanced simply by recruiting a sufficient number of physicians to the area even without introducing new specialties. Changes in retention can best be forecast as results of specific anticipated or planned changes in service capacity: new physicians, greater bed capacity if current capacity is overcrowded, added specialties, or new services.

In a recent case the method used to forecast the increased retention expected from adding a hospital to a suburban area predicted retention as a function of the bed and population ratio. Without the new hospital the area enjoyed a ratio of 1.67 beds per thousand population. Following the addition of the hospital, this ratio would increase to 1.88 (growing population diminished the ratio effect of the new facility). With a 45% retention level without the new hospital, this produced an estimate that retention would increase to $1.88 \div 1.67 \times 45\% = 50.7\%$.

Such a calculation was intended as a simple, objective approach to estimating retention. Because the new hospital would be in a previously unserved location, it would add to the accessibility as well as availability of care. For this reason, retention would probably increase to more than 50.7%. It is not possible to claim that an increase in the bed and population ratio would *cause* an increase in retention. Given the expected consequences of developing a new hospital, i.e., attracting more physicians to the area, providing a more convenient source of inpatient care, a significant increase in retention was confidently expected.

**Preference**

The extent to which any given hospital experiences use by a given service population is a function of the relative preference for hospitals in the area. This is no different, of course, from the fact that retention is a function of their relative preference for hospitals within the area versus elsewhere. The market shares enjoyed by hospitals within the same service area are subject to significant swings for purely psychographic reasons, however, where retention is more a function of service changes.

Preference by physicians is and will likely remain the most important determinant of a hospital's market share. This may be preference regarding which medical staff to belong to or which hospital to refer more patients to when multiple membership on medical staffs is the rule. Patients are undoubtedly exerting more influence on this latter form of preference than in the past, though by no means dominating choice.

Preference for individual hospitals is difficult to predict precisely because it is susceptible to significant short-term influence through effective marketing. Finding out why physicians prefer one hospital to another and responding accordingly can produce significant shifts in a short time. A scandal at one hospital, a nurses' strike, or a policy decision opposed by physicians can produce dramatic shifts to another hospital. Although development of medical campuses with doctors' office buildings adjacent to the hospital tends to produce greater loyalty in preference, it is no guarantee.

The best way to improve preference for a given hospital is to find out why physicians do not prefer it to begin with and act accordingly. Individual conversations with physicians are likely to work better than mailed questionnaires or even telephone interviews in this regard. Taking the time to meet with potential high admitters personally (the administrator or medical director is best) also communicates the extent of the hospital's interest and concern for each such physician.

**Inflow**

The number of patients coming to the hospital from elsewhere is typically forecast as a percentage of total admissions. Thus, if 20 percent of last year's admissions came from elsewhere, the tendency is to predict next year's local admissions, then divide them by 80 percent to estimate total admissions. In the short run this is probably not too bad, but in the long run it can be risky. To predict inflow, it is vital that the sources of such inflow and the reasons for it be identified and some thought given to whether *amounts* of inflow are likely to change.

Inflow should always be treated in terms of the number of admissions and patient days expected, not the percentage. If areas from which inflow comes are growing at a rapid rate while the natural service population is stagnating, the numbers of such patients and their proportion of the hospital's total are likely to increase. If the reverse is true or if new hospitals are being developed in such areas, inflow is likely to decrease in both absolute and relative terms.

To illustrate what can happen if inflow is treated as a constant percentage, imagine a case in which two areas are to be considered, the primary service area and everywhere else. To simplify the illustration, let us imagine that the two areas are islands (such as two of the Hawaiian Islands). Island A has a population of 100,000 while B claims 200,000. The use rate for island A residents is 1,000 inpatient days of care per person per year, while residents of B use 900. In the most recent year 50% of the residents of island A journeyed to B for care, while 20% of B residents traveled to A. With this information the flow of patients to each island can be calculated as follows:

- Residents of A

  —100,000 people × 1,000/1,000 patient days of care = 100,000 patient days
  —100,000 patient days × 50% outflow = 50,000 going to B
  —100,000 × 50% retention = 50,000 staying on A

- Residents of B

  —200,000 people × 900/1,000 patients days of care = 180,000 patients days
  —180,000 patient days × 20% outflow = 36,000 going to A
  —180,000 × 80% retention = 144,000 staying on B

- Hospitals on A. With 50,000 patient days staying on A and 36,000 coming in from B, the hospitals on A would enjoy 86,000 patient days, of which 36,000, or 41.86%, is inflow.

264 FORECASTING USE OF HEALTH SERVICES

- Hospitals on B. With 144,000 patient days staying on B and 50,000 coming in from A, hospitals on B would enjoy 194,000 patient days, of which 50,000, or 25.77%, is inflow.

In 10 years the population on B will decline to only 180,000 while A's population will grow to 150,000. Use rates will remain the same. Assuming that the patterns of flow remain constant, the use of care in the future can be calculated as follows:

- Residents of A

—150,000 people × 1.000 = 150,000 patient days of care used
—150,000 × 50% outflow = 75,000 patient days to B
—150,000 × 50% retention = 75,000 patient days staying on A

- Residents of B

—180,000 people × .900 = 162,000 patient days of care used
—162,000 × 20% outflow = 32,400 patient days to A
—162,000 × 80% retention = 129,600 patient days staying on B

If inflow were calculated as a constant proportion, A hospitals would anticipate it to be 41.86% of their total. With 75,000 patient days expected from retention, total utilization should be 75,000 ÷ (100% − 41.86%), or 75,000 ÷ .5814 = 128,999 total days. B hospitals would expect 129,600 retained patient days plus 25.77% inflow, so total days forecast would be 129,600 ÷ .7423 = 174,592 patient days.

Total patient days used by A and B residents would amount to 150,000 + 162,000 = 312,000. Total patient days forecast by A and B hospitals would amount to 128,999 + 174,592 = 303,591. Thus use of constant inflow percentages would result in losing almost 9,000 patient days that would not appear in either hospital's forecast. Moreover actual use of hospitals on A would be 75,000 retention + 32,400 = 107,400, although the forecast is 128,999, or 20 percent higher. Use of B hospitals would be 129,600 retention plus 75,000 inflow, or 204,600, although the forecast is 174,592, or 15 percent fewer patient days. Both sets of hospitals would be poorly prepared for actual utilization.

If inflow is a small amount and comes from a wide variety of places, as with a vacation area, it would be wisest not to predict much change at all unless a reason for it can be identified. If the hospital enjoyed 1,000 admissions this year from nonarea residents, it might better forecast 1,000 for next year and even the next 10 years rather than expect this number to behave exactly as its retention and market share do.

Once numerical values have been determined for each of these factors, the utilization forecast is simple. The service population is to be multiplied by the use rate, which is the product of admissions times average length of stay. The product of population times use rate is the total local utilization market available. Multiplying this figure times expected retention yields the extent to which all local hospitals will capture this market. Multiplying local capture times an individual hospital's market share yields its total expected utilization by service area residents. Adding in utilization by nonresidents produces the forecast of total utilization.

The following data and calculations illustrate this process. The data are

- Service area population = 150,000
- Forecast use rate = 150 admissions per thousand × 6.0 average length of stay = 900 patient days/1,000
- Forecast retention = 75% for all local facilities
- Forecast market share for hospital A = 55%
- Inflow to hospital A from beyond the service area forecast to be 5,000 patient days

150,000 × .900 = 135,000 patient days
135,000 × .75 = retained patient days in the area of 101,250
101,250 × .55 = 55,688 retained patient days at hospital A
55,688 + 5,000 inflow patient days = 60,688 total utilization

When applied to a new hospital, there is no specific past performance to go by. Moreover there is no simple quantitative model for anticipating the effect on retention, new inflow, or market share for a new facility. A survey of local physicians, perhaps supplemented by a survey of local residents, is probably as close to an objective approach as is available. Such surveys are suspect for a number of reasons, however. They tend to understate prospective utilization because they can survey only physicians who already practice in the area. This ignores the effect of a new hospital in attracting additional physicians. On the other hand it may overstate prospects because physicians may be reacting to what they hope the new hospital will be like, then be disappointed when it begins to operate.

The extent to which a new hospital increases retention and inflow is a function of its location: is it going to be developed in a previously unserved area or simply added to an existing complex of facilities; is it near the edge of the natural service area, hence close to people outside, or is it farther from outside areas than other existing facilities? Its inflow attraction is also a function of whether it offers unique services or develops effective marketing strategies for generating referrals. No substitute for informed judgment is available to forecast the use of a new hospital, and such a forecast should never be made passively.

## PRIMARY CARE CENTER FORECAST

To forecast use of a new primary care center, the same basic model is used as for hospital inpatient care. The natural service area is smaller in most cases. However, if the center is designed to serve commuters working in a business district instead of or in addition to local residents, the service population would cover where people work more than where they live. Otherwise the natural service area would tend to be circumscribed by a radius of no more than 30 minutes' travel and typically no more than 15 to 20. If most residents of the area walk or use public transportation, this might amount to a few square miles. If driving personal cars is the mode, then a substantially larger area would apply.

The service area for primary care is partly a function of existing and potential competition as well. In defining a service area, it is usually wiser to select a larger area and expect a smaller market share than to select a small area with a large share but much hard-to-predict inflow.

Because a primary care center serves patients directly, its market is patients rather than physicians. If it were a specialty ambulatory care program, this would not apply, and the techniques appropriate for predicting hospital utilization would work. For a primary care program the most important factor is whether it intends and expects to serve as the basic source of care for the population that it serves. A center providing episodic, backup care might expect to see its patients only an average of once a year, for example. One offering regular care could hope to average three or more visits per year in contrast.

Thus the use rate and market shares for a specific primary care center would depend on how it is able to position itself in the market, as a sporadic walk-in backup source of care or as the equivalent of a personal and family physician. It may well be that a given center serves in both ways, as a backup for some portion of its market and a regular source of care for the rest. If so, the proportions of each must be forecast in order to predict overall utilization.

Imagine, for example, that the natural market contains 50,000 people. Of these let us say that 80 percent tend to seek and use a personal physician and 20 percent use care episodically. A given primary care center should thus anticipate serving three separate market segments:

1. some portion of the 80 percent aligned market who choose the center as their primary source of care
2. the rest of that 80 percent who use other sources as their primary source but might use the center as a backup facility
3. The nonaligned who might choose the center for some of their use

The local market should normally be surveyed to determine present utilization levels, attitudes, and preferences. Populations served by hospital emergency rooms but concerned over high costs, impersonal treatment, or long waits could easily be attracted to an urgicenter or walk-in clinic program. Populations comfortable with their present physicians but wishing for after-hours care would suggest that the center adopt hours accordingly. The best basis for forecasting and, more importantly, influencing utilization of a new primary care program is good market research followed by responsive program design and implementation.

Each market segment should be forecast separately to develop numerical estimates of utilization. Starting with 50,000 people, we know that 40,000 will be aligned and 10,000 nonaligned. If the center can capture 20 percent of the aligned market and serve as their regular source of care, it might predict 8,000 people $\times$ 2.5 visits average per person = 20,000 visits per year. For the aligned who might only use the center sporadically, if it can capture 20 percent of this market, it might predict 32,000 people $\times$ 0.5 visits $\times$ .20 = 3,200 visits per year, substantially less than it expects from regular patients. If it can attract 20 percent of the nonaligned market, it might predict 10,000 $\times$ 2.0 visits $\times$ .20 = 400 additional visits. Its total would then be 20,000 + 3,200 + 4,000 = 27,200 visits per year.

## SUMMARY

Forecasting use of a new program is vital to determining whether and how to develop such a program. A specific provider's utilization is always a function of the total market for the service being provided and of the share of that market that the provider can capture. The total market is in turn a function of the need for the service, the perceptions and attitudes of those in need, and the types of alternative sources of care available.

Some new programs can be approached through an incidence and prevalence technique, examining those people currently requiring a given service and adding the numbers expected to develop such a need in the future.

Demand for kidney dialysis services is an excellent example of this situation, where incidence and prevalence virtually dictate utilization level and provider choice. The same approach works for forecasting enrollment levels in an HMO.

Inpatient care utilization in a new hospital is a much more conjectural challenge. The choices of both physicians and patients must be forecast well in advance, opening up all the uncertainties of human perceptions and behavior in the relatively distant future. Total market, retention, inflow, and the share of the new hospital must be forecast, then combined quantitatively to produce a forecast of its utilization. Because achieving a given utilization level is vital, and influencing such use is certainly possible, passive forecasting techniques should not be used in such cases.

For the faster-growing primary care center market, utilization need not be forecast quite so far in advance. Because individual patients and families are the sole determinants of such use, however, it is subject to even less predictable factors than either kidney dialysis or hospital inpatient care. A much more conscious marketing approach to both forecasting and influencing demand for such a center is called for than in either of the two previous examples.

---

**Annotated Bibliography**

**Folland, S.** "Predicting Hospital Market Shares." *Inquiry* 20, no. 1 (Spring 1983):34.
   Discusses the use of hospital characteristics to predict competitive market shares among hospitals in rural areas, concluding that bed size and distance are most useful predictive factors, but others count as well.

**Glasgow, J. et al.** "Strategy for Determining Need for Cardiovascular Surgical Services." *Public Health Reports* 91, no. 1 (January–February 1979):67.
   Examines population-based approaches to forecasting use of cardiovascular surgery, given incidence of heart disease.

**Metcalfe, V.** *Renal Disease Services Criteria and Standards.* Monograph. Seattle: University of Washington, 1976.
   Describes complex set of factors involved in forecasting dialysis demand; estimates incidence at 35 to 40 new cases per million people per year.

**Newhouse, J.** "Forecasting Demand and the Planning of Health Services." In *Systems Aspects of Health Planning,* edited by G. Bailey. New York: American Elsevier, 1975.
   Discusses the use of health status factors in forecasting use of health services.

**Platt, R.** "Planning for Dialysis and Transplantation Facilities." *Medical Care* 11, no. 3 (May–June 1973):201.
   Estimates incidence of cases at 60 per million per year times three treatments per week.

# Appendix

# Glossary

**ARIMA (Auto-Regressive-Integrated-Moving-Averages)**—a complex, computer-based forecasting technique that combines moving averages with autoregression in analyzing past data as a basis for extrapolating into the future.

**Accuracy**—how close a forecast of future reality comes to that reality when it happens, can only be determined as the future occurs.

**Analog Forecasting**—estimating future utilization based on similar experience in another time or place, i.e., treating some other experience as an analogy for the future.

**Autocorrelation**—a forecasting technique that is based on the correlation between utilization in one period and the utilization in *one* prior period.

**Autoregression**—A specific type of autocorrelation in which the correlation between utilization in different periods is expressed as a regression.

**Box-Jenkins**—a complicated, computer-based time series analysis technique that fully identifies patterns of past utilization as a basis for extrapolating into the future.

**Causal Forecasting**—forecasting that consciously incorporates objective data and subjective judgments regarding the factors influencing utilization.

**Confidence Interval**—a range of values within which there is a known statistical probability that the truth falls, if based on a sample of past data, or within which there is an estimated probability the future will fall, if based on a forecast.

**Consistency**—the extent to which past observations fit whatever underlying pattern is deemed to describe them.

**Correction Point**—a point in the lead time when a decision can be altered before implemented or a point in the duration of a decision when the decision can be modified if utilization forecasts are revised.

269

**Delphi**—a subjective forecasting technique that combines the independent estimates of a number of informed persons into either a consensus or mathematically averaged forecast.

**Demographics**—factual, objective information about people that may be useful in predicting their use of health services: age, sex, race, income, education, residence, health status, insurance coverage, for example.

**Dependent Variable**—any reality that depends on the measured or forecast state of some independent variable to be estimated or forecast; appears on the left-hand side of mathematical expressions.

**Duration**—the time over which a decision is effective, hence during which utilization patterns determine whether the decision was successful.

**Exponential Smoothing**—a forecasting technique that adjusts a forecast of utilization based on the discrepancy between a forecast of the most recent period and actual utilization for that period.

**Extrapolation**—a forecasting technique that graphically, mathematically, or statistically identifies a pattern in a number of periods of past utilization, then extends that pattern into the future to forecast utilization.

**_F_ Test**—a measure that indicates whether a good fit between a regression and observed utilization ($r^2$ value) might have occurred by chance.

**Forecast**—a reasonable estimate of future reality, based on examination of present or past reality together with judgment regarding how reality might change.

**Fourier Regression**—a cyclical regression based on trigonometric functions (sine and cosine) calculated from past utilization data.

**Independent Variable**—any measurable reality that is used as the basis for forecasting, on whose present or future state a utilization forecast depends; appears on the right-hand side of mathematical expressions.

**Inflow**—the numbers of people who are not residents of a defined service area but who obtain care from providers in the area.

**Innovation Adoption Curve**—a forecasting technique based on past patterns involving the gradual adoption of new ways of doing things, suggesting slow early growth followed by a period of rapid growth, then leveling to no growth.

**Intercept**—the beginning point or zero base for a trend, i.e., the point where a trend graphically or mathematically originates.

**Interventionist Forecasting**—any objective or subjective approach to forecasting that identifies and incorporates ways that the forecaster can influence future utilization in the forecast.

**Lead time**—the time between the point when a decision is made and when that decision is in operation, e.g., between deciding to build or expand a facility and opening that facility for business.

**Market Segment**—a specific subset of a population that differs from other subsets in a way significant to either forecasting or influencing their use of health services, e.g., by age, sex, race, or residence.

**Market Share**—the proportion of all local utilization (e.g., all patient days or visits) that any single provider is able to capture in a given period. Separate shares can be calculated for retention and inflow and by specific service categories.

**Moving Averages**—a forecasting technique that calculates the averages across two or more periods of past utilization as the basis for forecasting, rather than relying on the data from individual periods.

**Naive Forecasting**—forecasting that incorporates no attempt to understand the causes of utilization or factors that might alter utilization patterns.

**Normal Distribution**—the most common statistical frequency distribution characterizing the pattern of observations expected around the mean or average of all observations.

**Outflow**—the numbers or proportion of people in the local market or service area who leave the area for some service.

**Passive Forecasting**—any objective or subjective approach to forecasting that assumes that the forecaster has no way of influencing future utilization.

**Persistence**—the extent to which past patterns continue to characterize observations in the future.

**Precision**—how narrow the range of forecast reality or how wide the range of uncertainty that accompanies a forecast.

**Prediction**—a forecasting technique that identifies a relationship between past utilization and some other factors, then predicts utilization as a function of the other factors.

**Product Life Cycle**—a pattern of sales volume or consumer behavior found to characterize specific product and brand experience, with different patterns prevalent, depending on how new any given product is and when competing brands emerge.

**Projection**—a forecasting technique that identifies a pattern in past utilization data and projects that pattern into the future, whether or not the causes of that pattern are identified and understood.

**Prospection**—a forecasting technique that relies on what can be foreseen about the future and its impact on future utilization of health services, with or without any knowledge or analysis of past patterns.

**Psychographics**—subjective information reported by people regarding what they believe or how they feel about themselves, health services, or specific providers, that can be useful in forecasting how they will use specific services or providers: perceived health status, health awareness, image of providers, knowledge of symptoms, for example.

$r^2$—a measure of how much closer a regression based on past data comes to observed utilization than does the calculated mean value of such utilization; indicates how well the regression characterizes past utilization but does not predict how well it forecasts utilization.

**Regression**—a statistical forecasting technique that expresses utilization as a function of constant and coefficient values applied to past utilization (linear or autoregression) or to other factors (multiple regression).

**Retention**—the numbers or proportion of people in the local market or service area who stay in that area for service.

**Slope**—a measure of the amount of change involved in a trend expressed as units of utilization per time period.

**Standard Deviation**—a measure of the extent to which past observations vary around their mean.

**Standard Error**—a measure of the extent to which past observations vary around their underlying trend.

**Time Lagging**—a technique for analyzing past and forecasting future utilization that uses relationships between utilization and some causal factor measured in different periods.

**Time Series Analysis**—a forecasting technique that identifies, then extrapolates complex patterns of past utilization broken down into trend, cycles, and seasonal fluctuations.

# Index